T0198642

# Acupuncture
# Revolution

The Science and Healing Power
of Acupuncture

JANET HUMPHREY

BALBOA.
PRESS
A DIVISION OF HAY HOUSE

Balboa Press books may be ordered through booksellers or by contacting:

Balboa Press
A Division of Hay House
1663 Liberty Drive
Bloomington, IN 47403
www.balboapress.com
1 (877) 407-4847

Because of the dynamic nature of the Internet, any web addresses or links contained in this book may have changed since publication and may no longer be valid. The views expressed in this work are solely those of the author and do not necessarily reflect the views of the publisher, and the publisher hereby disclaims any responsibility for them.

The author of this book does not dispense medical advice or prescribe the use of any technique as a form of treatment for physical, emotional, or medical problems without the advice of a physician, either directly or indirectly. The intent of the author is only to offer information of a general nature to help you in your quest for physical, emotional and spiritual well-being. In the event you use any of the information in this book for yourself, which is your constitutional right, the author and the publisher assume no responsibility for your actions.

Print information available on the last page.

ISBN: 978-1-5043-3476-1 (sc)
ISBN: 978-1-5043-3478-5 (hc)
ISBN: 978-1-5043-3477-8 (e)

Library of Congress Control Number: 2015909453

Balboa Press rev. date: 8/11/2015

# WHAT PATIENTS ARE SAYING
# ABOUT ACUPUNCTURE
. . . . . . . . . . . . . . . . . . . . .

"Acupuncture has helped me in so many ways. I was at a point where I thought nothing would help relieve my chronic back and shoulder pain. I couldn't stand myself! Through acupuncture I finally found relief. I've also been able to use acupuncture to treat other musculoskeletal injuries enabling me to heal quicker and be back on my feet sooner. I've found if I now have regular preventative treatments I reduce the incidence of flare-ups, I feel more balanced and I'm generally happier (because I'm not in pain!). For me, acupuncture is part of a healthy lifestyle for my mind and body."

-Corey G.

"Acupuncture has fundamentally shifted the foundations in my life. What started with treatment for the excruciating pain associated with sciatic nerve stress eight years ago became, and remains, a pathway on my journey to self-healing. Not all acupuncturists are equally equipped to know the soul. I consider myself outstandingly fortunate. I see my acupuncturist on a weekly basis - disruptions to this routine occur, but are most unwelcome. At a basic level, I see her to manage life's stresses, pain from running and for general wellness. More fundamentally, acupuncture provides me with a window through which to contemplate and better understand that the root of pain and healing are one and the same. They require regular balancing of the life sustaining energy we all possess within to coexist and function optimally."

-Ingrid B.

"I was always resistant to the idea of acupuncture - not because I had any aversion to alternative therapies but because I was into so many I hesitated to add another commitment. I first encountered it directly when my husband was diagnosed with painful plantar fasciitis. His doctor gave him no hope and only offered one untenable suggestion - that my husband take some 30 painkillers a week. That clearly toxic proposition, the podiatrist said, might not even work. Instead of trying this course of action, which had a definite negative outcome and no certain positive one, my husband tried acupuncture. With one session, his pain was gone, and within a few more he was cured.

"When I developed neuroma in my feet following bad surgery, I similarly had nowhere to turn and went to my husband's acupuncturist. I was immediately hooked on the sense of well-being and relaxation, and, like my husband, my feet problems were easily cured by her needles with no bad side effects. I continued to get acupuncture long after the initial symptoms subsided.

"Around that time, we were trying to conceive our third child. It was a long shot considering I was over 40. My acupuncturist began to provide treatment for fertility. I got pregnant three times, and although I lost the first two pregnancies in the first trimester (likely a natural reaction to fetal abnormalities) I became pregnant again at 43 and delivered our third healthy son when I was nearly 44.

"Since then, acupuncture has continued to provide relief for my body, especially back pain which I suffered following a lull in treatments which was quickly cured when I resumed them. Most interestingly and perhaps surprisingly, it has opened my creative centers. As a writer, this is tremendously important, and a source of healing that only my acupuncturist, unique among any health professional I have ever seen, identified. I am forever grateful for her compassionate care, which has definitely transformed my life significantly for the better."

-Jessica J.

"Acupuncture has changed my life. Bold statement, I know. But it is the truth. I started receiving treatment about four years ago and I can't imagine my life without it. Of course, a wonderful acupuncturist makes all of the difference. I was initially amazed at how my chronic knee pain went away after one treatment. I was hooked! For me, the trigger point approach was fascinating and easily made me a believer – I could feel my body releasing. I think that is important in Western culture – we need to feel that something is working. Aside from targeted problem spots, I can also feel the overall benefits of my treatments. I maintain a regular acupuncture schedule because it simply puts my body back in balance. I also use acupuncture as a preventative measure – it's the first step I use if I'm feeling rundown and fearful I might be getting sick. It's a fantastic, natural alternative to medication."

-Michelle F.

"Acupuncture relieved the pain in my thumb joint from rheumatoid arthritis that made it hard to use my hand. After 5 years of trying different drugs that didn't work, my hand felt astonishingly better in just one acupuncture treatment. At the same time, it helped me feel more relaxed, helped ease my back pain, and perhaps more importantly, it made me feel connected and peaceful. This is part of the reason I keep coming back, for a sense of peace and thoughtfulness."

-Karen B.

"Acupuncture has changed my life. Whether is was to treat specific conditions like high blood pressure and digestion, or for general well-being and improved energy levels, I cannot imagine life without it."

-Fred S.

"As someone who has always believed that to maintain optimal health, we have to focus on both our physical and spiritual dimensions, I have used acupuncture as a modality over the past 15 years, not only as an adjunct to traditional medicine when I've been sick or injured, but as a "tune up" to bring me back in balance. During an acupuncture treatment, I actually feel energy (spirit) flowing throughout my body, which creates an immediate sense of calm and a natural high. Acupuncture cured my chronic sinusitis, and when my blood pressure became elevated a single acupuncture treatment restored it to normal. For those who've never tried acupuncture, I highly recommend it! Be open and don't worry about the "needles," it's really painless."

-Mary Louise H.


"Acupuncture has helped me in a myriad of ways. I initially tried acupuncture 11 years ago after suffering a severe leg break. My leg healed quickly and the treatments also helped with the emotional trauma of the accident. During my career on a Wall Street trading floor I could not have survived the day-to-day stresses without weekly acupuncture. And when faced with unexplained infertility, acupuncture sessions made me relax physically, mentally and spiritually, ensuring my first round of IVF was a success.

"Now, as a stay-at-home parent of a 7-year-old and a 5-year-old, acupuncture is more important than ever. It helps to balance, relax and focus me so I can be a happy, patient and loving parent.

"You can measure the benefits of acupuncture in your physical well-being but what I find the most fascinating and beneficial is the spiritual and emotional "rest" I receive from each session."

-Elizabeth R.

"Acupuncture has changed the course of my life—and not just because the treatments have helped me, but my own personal experience with these treatments inspired me to change my career path. From the moment I got on the table at my first appointment, I started asking a zillion questions about how and why needles were being placed where they were; how do you know where a point is located; why does a point in my foot make my head feel better; how do you get that muscle to twitch? Years later I have not stopped asking, and my fascination continues to grow. So much so that, two years ago, after nearly 15 years working in a career that I had thought I would be in for life, I made the most spontaneous, crazy, daunting, life-changing decision to-date, and went back to school to earn my Master of Science in Acupuncture. I have not regretted my decision for a single moment and the thought that I will be making people feel better every day through a modality that has healed so many of my own pains, kept my stress level in check and my body in balance and healthy, constantly puts a smile on my face. All of this, coupled with having an incredible acupuncturist and mentor to guide me, has cemented my belief in the benefits of this centuries-old art."

-Jamie F.

# DEDICATION

· · · · · · · · · · · · · · · · · · · ·

To all the scholars, teachers, researchers, scientists, clinicians and patients – past, present and future – who keep the art and science of healing alive,

And to my niece, Ruby Joan Liang Humphrey.

# TABLE OF CONTENTS

· · · · · · · · · · · · · · · · · · ·

# PREFACE

. . . . . . . . . . . . . . . . . . . .

"Sooner or later, everything old is new again."
—Stephen King, *The Colorado Kid*

Acupuncture is a rich tradition, one of profound depth and nuance that reveals itself in wondrous, surprising ways as you journey into it. One can devote a lifetime to the study and practice of acupuncture, gain mastery of its practice, and still feel that there is so much more to learn. Acupuncture takes you on a journey into awareness of life itself.

The *Acupuncture Revolution* is not a takeover of modern medicine by an ancient technique. It's an infusion of perspective and a reawakening to the true nature of healing in our medicine and in our lives. Acupuncture is a way to relieve pain, but it is also much more than that. As you relieve your pain with acupuncture, you touch into a sense of your own wholeness, and the potential for living a more complete and fulfilling life.

Every culture throughout history has had its own healing ways. Ours—contemporary scientific medicine—is the latest, but it surely won't be the last. Western medicine has strengths but it seems to have forgotten that healing is more than just keeping the body alive. The potential for healing is present in every moment; indeed, you can heal even as you die. Healing comes through our challenges, our pain, our losses, our sufferings, the small deaths woven into life—if we allow it.

Acupuncture is grounded in an appreciation for the arc of birth, growth, and death that's inherent in life. It recognizes the unity of body, mind, emotions, and spirit, and unlocks the potential for healing from within. It takes us deeper into what it means to be fully human in an interconnected world—within an even vaster interwoven universe.

This awareness can make all forms of medicine more effective—moving beyond just the elimination of symptoms to optimizing wellness at all levels, beyond prolonging life at all costs to living - and dying – in wholeness, integrity and contentment. It reminds us to treat the patient and not just the illness.

Most of the patients I see in my acupuncture practice are suffering from ailments that are the result of long-standing imbalances: pain, fatigue, chronic sinus congestion, allergies, infertility, digestive problems—conditions that can only be fully resolved by restoring the body's innate capacity for self-healing. Some patients are suffering from pain, anxiety or depression that can only be healed when they reconnect with their life's passion and let it guide their lives. This is healing from the level of "spirit."

When you go for acupuncture treatment, you receive much of what conventional medicine is not providing. There's a very personal approach. The acupuncturist spends time with you, asking questions like:

- What's your lifestyle?
- How do you eat?
- How do you sleep?
- Do you tend to feel warm or cold?
- What are your challenges?
- How are your relationships?
- Do you exercise?
- How do you like your work?
- Are you married or single?
- Do you have children?
- Did you have many infections as a child?
- What was happening in your life at the time your symptoms started?

The acupuncturist uses touch, feeling your areas of pain or dysfunction. When you feel that touch, there is a deep experience of being understood and recognized. This builds trust and it's reassuring. It affirms your sense of what is happening in your own body, and begins to bring your awareness more deeply to its needs. The treatment itself usually gives you an immediate experience of improvement. If you came in with pain, your pain is reduced or eliminated. You tend to feel relaxed beyond all expectations and very uplifted.

Acupuncture has become popularly promoted for quitting smoking and for weight loss. Many people ask if it works. Yes, it does, but not in the way you'd imagine. It's not like taking a pill and you magically quit smoking or lose weight. It involves balancing you, activating your body's own healing abilities, normalizing blood sugar, improving metabolism, relieving anxiety and depression, and reducing unhealthy cravings, thereby supporting you in your efforts to quit smoking and lose weight.

In our symptom-oriented medical culture, acupuncture has been highlighted for its ability to relieve pain and other unwanted symptoms. It does this, and much more. Acupuncture treats the source of your symptoms, helping your body heal itself, and restores balance even *before* symptoms arise. A Chinese proverb says, "Don't wait until you're thirsty to dig a well." Acupuncture can be used to keep you healthy in the first place.

In acupuncture diagnosis, we rely upon the powers of observation, using touch and all of our senses to understand the root cause of symptoms. Through my observations—reading the pulse, tongue, and other signs of the body—I'm able to understand a great deal about a patient's imbalances. Presented with the insights that these observations provide, people often ask, "Are you psychic?" but I'm just reading the signs the body is showing.

One of the things we've sacrificed in modern Western medicine is this ability for physicians to "read the body." Instead, our doctors are being taught to order scans and to read the images and printouts on paper. These results, while valuable, are also very linear and generally fail to reveal the source of a patient's ailment. When that is the case, resolving the ailment in a truly healing way becomes difficult, if not impossible. Acupuncture still uses these powers of observation in understanding the patient, and then it accesses the body's own self-healing abilities in order to restore health.

In my clinical profession, as an acupuncturist, I am often asked how acupuncture works and what conditions it treats. Most people aren't looking for in-depth training in the philosophy of traditional Chinese medicine, but instead want to know something about where it comes from and how it can help them. The idea of placing needles in points around the body to heal is so foreign, and patients are looking for a way to understand it. To help with this, we look to science.

Scientific studies are underway to elucidate how acupuncture works. We have a lot of evidence about its effects but no comprehensive explanations yet. One of the challenges in studying acupuncture is the tendency to boil it down to its most mechanical aspect—needle insertion—and measure effects in the body. This may provide misleading results. Acupuncture's theoretical context provides the key to its effective use. Not every patient with the same symptom requires the same acupuncture treatment. Needling technique can be separated from the theory and done in isolation, but it won't yield the same results. An acupuncturist must understand acupuncture on its own terms to perform it well. This is the "secret ingredient" in the recipe.

Throughout history, new ideas and observations have frequently preceded their scientific validation. True science ideally maintains an open-minded attitude and goes about testing and trying to understand perceived phenomena, such as acupuncture's healing effects. However, there are those who misapprehend science and take both its method and its existing understanding as dogma—something that repels change and reflexively refutes all that seems inconsistent with what is currently known.

The Internet, in particular, is disproportionately fraught with the shouting objections of naysayers who seem to have a suspiciously strong need to make acupuncture, as well as other complementary therapies, wrong and invalid. There is anger and hyperbole in their writings, and they give you the feeling of a bully shouting you down. I haven't discerned what motivates them, but while they're busy shouting, many people are getting better with these therapies and earnestly wanting to understand how they work.

*Does acupuncture replace conventional medicine?* No, it does not. Given the advances in Western medical science, acupuncture is no longer meant to be a comprehensive medical system on its own. Both systems can exist side-by-side and work together. Each provides something different. They need not compete or, alternatively, become homogenized into one.

*Does acupuncture work?* As an acupuncturist for nearly three decades now, I can tell you for sure that people are getting better from using it. I have had the most avowed skeptics turn into enthusiasts within an hour—having arrived with severe pain, they emerge from treatment nearly pain-free—something they never expected, and were quite certain was impossible. As an academically trained scientist who has worked as a biochemist and molecular biologist, I can say that the scientific research to-date is intriguing but equivocal. There are certainly data to demonstrate acupuncture's effects and efficacy. There are also data that are ambiguous and inconclusive, or at times apparently disproving acupuncture's effects. The design of scientific studies may at times be deeply flawed, as we struggle to create controls for a treatment whose mechanism we do not understand. We are, as yet, far from consensus on *how* acupuncture works. Research is ongoing. As we await results of that research, healing acupuncture treatments are also ongoing.

There is no way to do justice to the study of acupuncture and its tradition in a book of this kind—an introduction, a presentation of the face of acupuncture in today's world, to patients of today. The goal is to provide you with a bridge to this way of potential healing, an entryway into it that will allow you to try it for yourself. Once you've done that, your experience will be your guide, and your own unlocked inner resources will inform and amaze you. There are many great books that take you deeper into the philosophy of acupuncture, offering you further opportunities to access its wisdom for your life's healing journey.

The key to healing lies in the empowerment of the patient with knowledge. That includes understanding the body's integrative healing nature, and how you can actively generate health at every stage of life. This awareness is at the heart of acupuncture healing. It can also empower you to live and use all forms of medicine in the best way possible. In this book, I hope to give you an understanding of acupuncture's applications and its mechanisms in a way that allows you to use it most effectively along with other treatments for your health.

# AUTHOR'S NOTE

· · · · · · · · · · · · · · · · · · · ·

In trying to answer the questions about acupuncture that I hear most often in my clinical practice, I've organized this material in a way that I hope will be most useful to you. To do this, I've made choices about translation of Chinese terminology as well as presentation of patient treatments that bear a brief explanation.

The case histories are organized by age and gender to make it easier for readers to access material they will find relevant. These are, in a sense, artificial delineations; all readers can find pertinent healing stories within any of these sections. I've also selected patient profiles that are typical of those I often see in my practice. I've tried to do them justice and show you how a symptom like back pain can lead into discovery of unresolved grief or other root causes of which you, as a patient, may not be aware, and how acupuncture healing encompasses these as well. There are multiple subtle depths of healing touched within patient treatments that are beyond the scope of this book; for this reason, I have not gone into those details. In describing acupuncture encounters, patients' names and identifying details have been changed to protect their privacy.

The scientific studies are specifically notated and referenced to their respective sources. References used for general information within the rest of the book are listed at the end.

In explaining acupuncture, traditional Chinese medical terminology is used. Many of these terms have no direct translation into English; other terms are translated into English words that denote concepts very different from what is usually meant in English usage. In seeking a clear but simple way to handle this, I have chosen to use the following system throughout this book.

For terms that are unique to Chinese medicine and relatively well-recognized and widely used, I have kept the pinyin translation using lower case. These include *qi* (pronounced "chi"), *yin, yang, shen, jing*, and *jin ye*.

For terms that are translated into English where the Chinese term and its English equivalent have different meanings, I have taken two directions:

- In cases where confusion can easily arise for the reader, I have capitalized the English translation. These terms include the Chinese concept of Blood and the names of the organs: Heart, Liver, Kidney, Lung, Spleen, Stomach, Bladder, Gallbladder, Small Intestine, Large Intestine, Pericardium and Triple Heater.
- In cases where the context makes it easy to differentiate the Chinese meaning from the conventional English meaning, I have kept the English translation in lower case. These terms include pathogenic factors such as wind, dampness, heat, cold, and dryness and the elements of fire, earth, metal, water and wood.

I have used the term "acupuncture" in the broadest sense to encompass the entire system of diagnosis and treatment within traditional Chinese medicine apart from herbal medicine. In scientific research, this terminology must be used with much greater specificity for accuracy and precision. For example, using pressure on an acupuncture point is different from using a needle; using a needle and stimulating it manually is different from using electrical stimulation—and has different measurable effects. Burning warming herbs over an acupuncture point—the practice known as "moxibustion," is different from needle insertion. Diagnosis—taking the pulse and palpating body points—is itself altogether different from needling, though it may ultimately be found to have therapeutic effects in and of itself, as may the therapeutic conversational interaction with the patient. For ease of communication in the context of a book for lay readers, I have subsumed all of these elements under the term "acupuncture." Because the term "acupuncture point" is frequently used in this book, I have often abbreviated it to the commonly used alternate term, "acupoint," and these two terms are interchangeable.

In summarizing clinical patient evaluations, I have simplified the acupuncture diagnosis for the lay reader instead of listing the complete differential diagnosis as it would appear in treatment notes or in presentations to acupuncturists.

In reporting on scientific studies of acupuncture, I have included research that uses animal models for testing, specifically rats, mice, rabbits, cats and dogs. The scientific community has established its own ethical guidelines for use of animals in research, and the research reports always note their adherence to these guidelines in conducting these studies. I have very mixed feelings about the use of animals in research. While I recognize that animal modeling has facilitated research leading to breakthroughs in medicine and scientific knowledge—understanding that may go on to save many human lives—I still regret that we live in a world where animals are used in this way. I had considered avoiding drawing upon research studies based on animal modeling, but decided to include them. If these animals were sacrificed to further our scientific knowledge, at least that knowledge can be shared and put to its best use. I hope that in the future we are able to come up with alternative forms of research that do not involve the use of animal models.

I wish to thank Robin Bisland for her editorial contributions, Tom Starace for his illustrations, Sasha Illingworth for her cover design, and Kerry Kehoe for her photography. Thanks to Ruchi Misra and Ellen Ellis, L.Ac. for taking the time to review the manuscript and offer their insightful feedback and wisdom.

All of my teachers – too many to name – have contributed to my learning both in science and acupuncture healing. Special mention is due to Robert Zeiger, L.Ac., OMD, acupuncturist and herbalist, who took me on as a young apprentice and gave of his knowledge so generously; Robert Engel, Ph.D., who gave me the eyes with which to see the natural world; and John Barnes, P.T., who introduced me to fascia and led me through the door of healing in the most profound way.

I also wish to thank my patients, who have honored me with their trust and taught me so much.

This book includes aspects of the science, history, and benefits of acupuncture, and how to use it along with conventional medicine. You are invited to jump around and read whatever interests you. Some people will be drawn to the science, and others to the case histories. Yet others will want to know more about acupuncture's history. Feel free to use the back-of-the-book index to find conditions that interest you most and go straight to them. For topics that pique your interest, the references will provide leads to outstanding books that will take you deeper. I want this book to be useful to you in whatever way works best for you.

# CHAPTER ONE

· · · · · · · · · · · · · · · · · · · ·

# My Introduction to Acupuncture

"In all affairs it's a healthy thing now and then to hang a question mark on the things you have long taken for granted."
—Bertrand Russell

Acupuncture first caught my attention when I was conducting scientific research at the University of California, while on leave from a doctoral program in nutritional biochemistry at Cornell University. Finding myself with stubborn sinus congestion and a cough that medical treatment had not helped, I thought I'd give acupuncture a try.

My local acupuncturist's office was in a converted barn in the backyard of her home. Inside, I smelled the rich and earthy aromas of Chinese herbs mingling. A wall was lined with shelves that held jars of dried herbs and tablets. The space was cozy, with beds for treatment in several rooms. It felt homey and warm—not like your typical doctor's office.

I told the acupuncturist my symptoms. She felt my pulse on both wrists, looked at my tongue, and inserted some acupuncture needles in my arms and legs. I'd simply rolled up my sleeves and pant legs so she could reach these areas. After placing the fine needles – I barely felt them being inserted – she handed me some tissues and asked cryptically, "Is it worth it?" Then she left the room, leaving me with a little bell to ring if I needed her.

I immediately relaxed and felt the tension leave my body. It was a calm, comfortable feeling. Within a few minutes, I began to cry. I didn't see that coming. During the previous year, there had been a lot of changes in my life: my father had died and I'd moved across the country, away from friends and family, to a new town and job.

As my body relaxed, I felt a kind of relief and sadness mixed together. I wondered how the acupuncturist knew I would need those tissues when I hadn't even been aware of it myself. Later, I learned about Chinese pulse reading and how much it can reveal about a person's condition, including stress, pent-up sadness, and anxiety as well as purely physical problems. This must have been how she knew.

By the time she returned to the room, the sadness had passed and I was in an even deeper state of relaxation, almost like sleep but still awake. My breathing was deep and easy, and my sinuses felt clear. I told her about the tears, and she gave me a knowing smile as she rechecked my pulse. She never explained it to me, but I felt better. She sent me home with a bag of herbs to brew into a medicinal tea.

After this visit, my cough and sinuses cleared up rapidly. It had been an impressive experience; the acupuncture had healed me, but I had no idea how. Not only had my physical symptoms resolved, but it seemed as if my emotions and life situation had somehow been treated as well. This intrigued me, and I continued to return for more treatments. Over the next few years, the treatments worked again and again. Eventually, at my acupuncturist's urging, I began to consider studying acupuncture myself.

After my cough and sinusitis cleared up, you may wonder why I continued returning for acupuncture treatment. Well, I was only in my mid-20s but I'd burned myself out. As I discovered later, and as you'll see in the patient healing stories, this is typical of people in their 20s. Having blazed through college burning the candle at both ends—studying hard and living to the max (sleep? what sleep?), going to graduate school, starting a new job and then another new job, moving far from home—I was having a blast. However, my body wasn't quite as enthusiastic. My adrenals were shot and I was tired all the time. Not just tired: if I blinked at

> *It had been an impressive experience; the acupuncture had healed me, but I had no idea how. Not only had my physical symptoms resolved, but it seemed as if my emotions and life situation had somehow been treated as well.*

work, I ran the risk of falling asleep while standing. There were dizzy spells. I was a burn-out case. That's why I returned for acupuncture treatments over the next two years.

In addition to giving me treatments, my acupuncturist gave me dried herbs to cook into a medicinal tea. She told me to add chicken bones to the brew because, she said, I was so depleted that I needed the "yang" nourishment that plant food couldn't give me. Though I was a vegetarian, I followed her instructions. When I told her I usually had oatmeal or cereal for breakfast, she told me to add two eggs and a piece of toast! It sounded like too much food. I didn't even have much of an appetite (which, as it turned out, was another sign of my depletion). I was perplexed. I had no idea how drained I was, but little by little, as I followed her instructions and received acupuncture treatments, I came to understand it.

It took me two years to get my full strength back. During that time, if I tried to go back to my old ways of overdoing it, my energy would immediately crash. This is adrenal exhaustion. In a way, it's good that it took two years to heal, because it took that long to rehabilitate my habit of overwork and living without tending to my own body's needs.

This is my story, but it's probably your story too. Almost everyone I meet, and everyone I treat with acupuncture, lives in a state of overdoing it, without giving enough healing care and restoration to their own body. It's our culture. And it's very much at the root of our disease. I know how hard it is to change that pattern, but you must. Most people wait until they hit the wall to make a change. Finally, your body "makes you an offer you can't refuse." You reach down to pick up a piece of paper and your back goes out. You get the flu and can't get out of bed for a month. You start waking up with panic attacks. These are all your body's way of saying, "Enough, I can't go on like this." Try to take steps to heal before you reach that point. Acupuncture is a potent healing method to restore your worn-out body, mind and spirit, and thereby heal what ails you.

*How does acupuncture work?* What is its scientific basis? As a biochemist turned acupuncturist, I should be able to answer these questions easily. But, I don't actually know the answers. No one does. Scientists, physicians, and clinical acupuncturists are researching the elusive mechanisms of acupuncture. We have a lot of intriguing data and proof of its effects, but no comprehensive explanation for how the placement of needles in different parts of the body helps with the healing process.

When I began studying acupuncture, it was hard to get my head around a foreign technique that had absolutely no basis in modern science. But over the years I've been repeatedly impressed by how effective it is. Not only does acupuncture relieve pain, but it also treats a range of internal diseases such as asthma, acid reflux, high blood pressure, irritable bowel syndrome, insomnia, anxiety, and vertigo. And on top of that, it provides an indescribable feeling of well-being that takes the edge off the stress of life—and who couldn't use some of that these days?

There are those who doubt that acupuncture works at all, and believe it's nothing more than snake oil medicine with a big dose of the placebo effect—that patients feel better solely because they believe the treatment will help them. This is unlikely, however, because although we don't yet know precisely how acupuncture works, studies that control for this effect have shown distinct physical results. Using blood tests to measure neurotransmitters, hormones, and natural painkillers as well as brain imaging, scientists have shown that acupuncture causes measurable changes in the body's physiology.[1] This is even true in animals, where the expectation of acupuncture "working" plays no part at all.

Others don't believe that sticking a needle in specific locations in the body can provoke therapeutic changes, as acupuncture contends. However, evidence suggests that different replicable effects can be measured depending on where and how the needle is placed, indicating that point specificity matters.[2] Other studies, using groups of people suffering from the same condition, such as low back pain or high blood pressure, validate acupuncture's therapeutic effects.[3]

Because science hasn't yet provided a full explanation, acupuncture's supporters and critics

> *Using blood tests to measure neurotransmitters, hormones, and natural painkillers as well as brain imaging, scientists have shown that acupuncture causes measurable changes in the body's physiology.*

alike can make similarly compelling arguments to bolster their cases. Until we have solid scientific evidence, we're still navigating by long tradition, opinion, and anecdotal evidence. Firsthand accounts from people whom acupuncture has helped seem at least partly responsible for the practice's growing popularity. When you hear that your colleague's migraines were relieved using acupuncture, or your cousin's back pain went away, you begin to wonder if it can help you with your neck pain, anxiety, or allergies. And you're more likely to try it yourself.

Interestingly, Western medical treatments also are often difficult to explain. We call them scientific because they involve technology, seem objective and precise, and are backed by scientific research. That's often the case. However, medications are frequently given for conditions simply because they've been observed to work, not because we understand their mechanisms of action. Many off-label uses of drugs fall into this category. By the same token, doctors may test an unproven procedure on a patient, and if it works, then that procedure may become more widely used and eventually made the focus of a study. So even the medicine that we consider to be scientific isn't entirely so. I point this out not to discredit Western medicine, but simply to show that in any medical system, the science—and its proofs—often comes after the treatment has been shown to work.

## Understanding Acupuncture

By investigating the science behind the time-tested technique of acupuncture, we're attempting to build a major new bridge between two dissimilar worlds. Acupuncture was developed in ancient China more than two thousand years ago in a culture, a period, and through a language completely foreign to contemporary Western sensibilities.

We tend to assume that today we're more knowledgeable and advanced, and that a Chinese physician from ancient times would have been too primitive and uninformed to understand health and medicine. We disdain him before we even meet him; we discount all that came before as part of an ignorant past. We may soon learn that this doctor from ancient times understood a lot more than we could have imagined.

As a patient, I overcame my own skepticism because acupuncture made me feel better, and I knew from experience that it was working. It seemed to generate health from the inside out. But as a scientist, I wanted to know how it worked and was loathe to admit to my colleagues that I took it seriously—to the point of studying it.

At the time, there was no science to explain acupuncture. To make matters worse, the language used to explain it sounded absolutely primitive. A common cold was described as an attack of "evil wind," a urinary tract infection was described as "damp heat in the lower burner," while nausea and vomiting were described as "counterflow *qi*."

When I took the leap into studying acupuncture, I struggled with this for a long time. And yet, I knew I'd encountered a healing system that could both prevent and cure many kinds of illness effectively. In addition to acupuncture, the

> *As a patient, I overcame my own skepticism because acupuncture made me feel better, and I knew from experience that it was working. It seemed to generate health from the inside out. But as a scientist, I wanted to know how it worked and was loathe to admit to my colleagues that I took it seriously—to the point of studying it.*

system of Chinese medicine includes herbal medicine as well as dietary and lifestyle remedies.

If I waited for science to explain how acupuncture worked, I reasoned, I'd probably wait a lifetime. I prize scientific research but what drew me to science in the first place was health and healing. If I stayed in the lab, I might spend decades understanding the function of a single enzyme or a section of DNA. As interesting and important as such research is, I chose instead to work with a system that helped people get better and improve their quality of life in real time.

## Can Valid Treatment Come from Invalid Concepts?

I now understand that Chinese disease patterns describe something real and treatable, even though they may seem inconsistent with our scientific understanding of the body. At some point, we may be able to translate these patterns into the language of Western anatomy and physiology, and understand precisely what they are describing. To a certain extent this is taking place already, as acupuncturists compare their observations to Western medical diagnoses.[4] This conversation is taking place more in the acupuncture community than in the scientific community, where the focus is more on testing the effects of acupuncture itself.

Historical documentation suggests that demonology played an extensive role in the concept of health and illness in ancient China. This grew out of earlier shamanic traditions that understood illness as an affliction sent by demons or displeased ancestors. The "treatment" included spells and rituals to appease the ancestors or cast out the demons.

If the fundamental concepts of ancient Chinese medicine were originally associated with demonology and magic, can they be valid in medical treatment? Could there be some thread that connects the magic with the science? This is what acupuncture research is trying to discover. Perhaps the thread will turn out to be the observation of natural phenomena, described in the past as demons and more recently as germs, for example. Although the explanations change, the underlying observations might be rooted in something more permanent and true. Even today, science exists for us alongside non-scientific beliefs that arise from a human yearning to understand the subtle forces at work in our lives that we cannot yet explain.

> *If the fundamental concepts of ancient Chinese medicine were originally associated with demonology and magic, can they be valid in medical treatment?*

In some respects, ancient Chinese acupuncturists may have better understood the workings of the human body in health and illness than we do today. They grasped its nuances and the interrelationships among systems, and how to treat them effectively. Ancient Chinese doctors looked at the body through a different lens than we do, using metaphors from nature and society to describe its functions. It's not that they weren't aware of specific organs; the ancient Chinese had opened the body in surgery— contrary to legend that it was taboo and therefore to be avoided—and they knew a great deal about the shape, size, placement and functions of each of the organs.[5] However, they combined this knowledge with other observations and—using the tools they had at hand—emphasized the body's physiological workings in their medicine.

We can now identify specific organ functions and measure body chemistry in ways unknown to ancient Chinese physicians. Yet, despite its strengths, our scientific approach tends to be reductionist—breaking things down to their smallest parts and seeing them in isolation from one another. We are not good at understanding the body's integrity—how all of its parts work together as one whole to support health and healing.

The use of metaphor to describe the body's functions, along with the ability to see things from several different perspectives at once, is inherent in acupuncture healing. In my early acupuncture studies, I apprenticed with an accomplished acupuncturist who had been practicing for many years. I watched as he diagnosed and treated patient after patient. Just when I thought I understood what he was doing and could anticipate how he would treat the next patient, he would do something completely different, and that approach worked as well. How did I assess that it "worked"? A patient with neck pain dramatically increased her range of motion immediately after the selected points were needled. I felt the release of muscle tension with my own hands and heard the patient report that the pain in the affected area had decreased. In addition, palpation of the Chinese pulses on the wrists revealed significant changes, corresponding to changes inside the body.

> *The use of metaphor to describe the body's functions, along with the ability to see things from several different perspectives at once, is inherent in acupuncture healing.*

In acupuncture, there are many ways to achieve healing, and no two acupuncturists may treat in exactly the same way. In this respect, acupuncture is an art as well as a science. As you will see, this is one of the reasons why it can be so challenging to design well-controlled scientific studies to validate its effects.

The growth of acupuncture in the United States began at a time when we were beginning to recognize some of the disadvantages of Western medicine. As a teenager in the 1970s, I was aware, watching some of my own family members, that doctors prescribed drugs that only put a band-aid on the symptom, without resolving the underlying condition. The side effects of one drug often led to the prescription of additional drugs. Patients were not infrequently misdiagnosed or mistreated, sometimes with disastrous results. There was a growing inclination at that time, and for me personally, to seek systems of healing aimed at restoring balance and regaining true health from the inside out.

Most people who come for acupuncture for the first time aren't sure what to expect. They have come because Western medicine has let them down, or they're looking for a more holistic treatment, or they're giving acupuncture a last-ditch try before submitting to a more drastic medical treatment, such as surgery. They want to understand how acupuncture works, and how to use it for their health. *Is it compatible with Western medicine, and if so, how?* Since gaining a foothold in the United States in the 1970s, acupuncture has continued to become established as an accepted method of treatment. Many physicians now recommend it to their patients.

Patients often assume that as an acupuncturist, I only support the use of "natural" medicine and oppose the use of Western medicine. They are surprised when I ask, "Have you considered surgery for this condition?" or "Have you had blood tests done to diagnose this?" While our medical system is less than perfect, it is also an invaluable approach to diagnosis and healing when we use it wisely.

In the chapters that follow, I hope to share with you "just enough" of the history and theory of acupuncture to demystify it. I will provide you with some of the latest scientific research on acupuncture's effects and its use in treatment for common conditions including pain, high blood pressure, and diabetes, among others. I will discuss what we know and don't know about how acupuncture really works, with illustrative case histories to show you how it's being used today, how it can help you, and how you can use it in conjunction with conventional Western medicine to optimize your overall health and well-being.

# CHAPTER TWO

· · · · · · · · · · · · · · · · · · · · ·

# How Acupuncture Heals

"The body can become a point of access into the realm of Being."
—Eckhart Tolle, *The Power of Now*

When I attended my first acupuncture classes, listening to introductory lectures on acupuncture theory, I was simply embarrassed for the instructors. They were talking about "wind" and "dampness" as causes of disease, and imbalances of "yin and yang" stirring up problems that led to illness. This seemed not only to be primitive thinking, but just wrong, based on imaginary concepts. Everyone knows that tuberculosis is caused by a bacterium and not by an imbalance of yin and yang, right? But the instructor showed us on the white board its progression, involving yin and yang, and ending with "this guy's dead!" Students took notes furiously while I wondered how on earth anything good could possibly come of this.

As I came to understand what was signified by the Chinese terms for illness, I began to see their validity. Far from being simplistic and primitive, these terms and concepts conveyed a sophisticated awareness of health and illness. When properly understood, it becomes clear how concepts such as yin and yang actually work as a highly effective system to guide treatment with acupuncture.

We have no language to accurately describe the concepts used by acupuncture in English. That's because its way of thinking and understanding of health is so different from ours. So we try to translate the Chinese language into terms we can understand, but it's not easy to do. This is why we still resort to using the Chinese terminology like *qi*, *yin* and *yang*. In my own practice, I use a lot of imagery to express my findings, because getting an education in Chinese medical theory is a project in itself, and Western medical terminology doesn't capture it at all. In time, perhaps we'll develop a third language through which these valuable healing concepts from ancient China can be properly described in English.

In the meantime, I'm going to give you a brief introduction to Chinese medical thinking, its main concepts and terminology, and an overview of acupuncture styles, including recent developments.

## Lost in Translation: Using Metaphor in Diagnosis and Treatment

Acupuncture, and all of Chinese medicine, invokes the use of metaphor. Yin/yang and the five elements are metaphors used in diagnosis and treatment. They are known as *systems of correspondences*. Using these two systems, everything in the natural world, and in the human body, can be categorized in relationship to every other thing. In its pure form, acupuncture is done completely within this context, without concern for modern anatomy and physiology.

This is where our contemporary understanding tends to break down. Either we discard the whole system as invalid or we struggle to translate these metaphorical systems directly into anatomy and physiology as we know it, and invariably fail to do so. It is difficult to find a one-to-one equivalent between the Chinese and Western concepts. The human body in Chinese medicine is seen through a completely different lens than in Western medicine.

We may never enjoy the satisfaction of finding exact equivalents for Chinese medical terminology in our own system. What we can reasonably expect to measure are the precise anatomical and physiological effects of acupuncture in the body. Bear in mind that we can only measure what we know. Our research is limited by the way we frame it. We like to believe that our knowledge is comprehensive, but even relatively recent scientific history proves otherwise.[1] We are encountering the limits of our previous knowledge with some regularity, and altering our theories accordingly. If you're looking for a buried treasure in the front yard, but it's actually in the back yard, you can dig forever and you will never find it. Likewise, if we seek to measure acupuncture's points and its effects by looking in the wrong place, the wrong way, or with the wrong instruments, we may not find them, although they are there. Let's take a closer look at how acupuncture views health through metaphor.

## Yin and Yang

We hear these terms a lot these days, but what do they really mean? In ancient China, all of creation was seen as a dual motive force that arose from the undifferentiated primary state. These two forces were designated as "yin" and "yang," respectively. They are interrelated and inseparable, and through their interaction all of life springs forth.

Fundamentally, yin is interpreted as "shady" and yang as "sunny," drawing upon the image of two sides of a hill, one illuminated by sunlight and the other in darkness. Because they are the primal forces behind all existence, everything in the universe can be attributed with qualities that correspond to either yin or yang. Yin is darkness, substance, cold, internal, feminine; yang is light, air, heat, external, masculine. They are not fixed identities but are always seen in dynamic interdependent relationships. In addition, something that is yin can be yang in relation to something else, and vice versa.

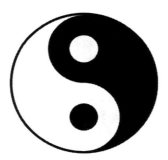

Yin (dark) and Yang (light) are balanced and interconnected. They represent the essential forces supporting health and all of life.

The yin/yang symbol is familiar to many of us. It depicts yin (dark) and yang (light) contained in equal balance within the whole, a circle. What are those two inner circles? Inside of the dark yin is a circle of light: yang; and inside the light yang is a circle of dark: yin. This reflects a hologram of yin held within yang, and yang within yin, inextricably connected in all of life. Indeed, the separation of yin and yang in the body, a change that can be felt in the pulse, indicates imminent death.

The forces of yin and yang are constantly in flux both in nature and in the body. We can see this in the change of night into day, spring to summer to fall to winter, and birth to maturity to old age and death. In the human body, these principles are at play at every level. Using this paradigm, every part of the body, mind, and spirit can be understood in terms of the interaction between yin and yang. Every organ and bodily function can be attributed with yin or yang qualities. In the most general sense, yin is more "solid" and substantial, taking the form of organs and fluids in the body, while yang is more ethereal, less substantial, correlated with movement and function. Yin might be seen as our anatomy, and yang as our physiology.

The acupuncture points and meridians are seen as repositories of yin or yang, able to restore balance, given the right stimulation. The acupuncturist looks for manifestations of imbalance through signs and symptoms. Once these imbalances are identified, acupuncture treatment is given to restore harmony between the fundamental forces of yin and yang. On a basic level, it's as simple as that. But to become adept in this system of diagnosis and treatment, refined skills of observation are required. Understanding how to read the body's signs in terms of yin and yang, and knowing the treatment method to restore balance, is essential.

An extension of the yin and yang system known as *the eight principles* is used clinically to identify *patterns of disharmony* in the body. The eight principles are:

- Yin and yang;
- Cold and heat;
- Interior and exterior;
- Deficiency and excess.

Once identified, the *patterns of disharmony* direct the acupuncturist to treatment principles, and the specific acupuncture points to use for healing the patient.

Sometimes, when people first come for acupuncture they ask, "Am I yin or yang?" Or sometimes they've been told that their yin is excessive, or their yang is weak. It's not really that fixed. Each of us reflects a dynamic interplay between the yin and yang forces within us, which are ever-changing. The key to effective acupuncture treatment, and to health, lies in promoting balance between these two forces. Identifying patterns of imbalance serves to direct treatment and lifestyle, and is never a fixed diagnosis.

## The Five Elements

The Five Elements can be seen as a further elaboration of yin and yang into more concrete components. These are described by elements observed in the manifest world: fire, earth, metal, water, and wood.

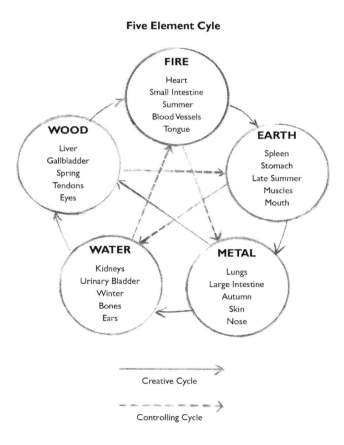

**Five Element Cyle**

The five elements cycle represents aspects of the body and the natural world, and the ways they support and balance one another.

Just as with yin and yang, each of the five elements has numerous correspondences. Earth corresponds to the Spleen and Stomach organ systems, to late summer season, and to worry, pensiveness, the color yellow, dampness, a singing tone of voice; whereas wood corresponds to the Liver and Gall Bladder organ systems, to spring, anger, frustration, the color green, wind, and a shouting tone of voice. These correspondences are diagnostic indicators that allow the acupuncturist to identify which systems are out of balance, and this leads to the choice of treatment. For example, if a patient craves sweets, the earth element (Spleen) may be imbalanced. If anger is excessive, the wood element (Liver) may be imbalanced. Treatment is aimed at bringing all the elements back into healthy balance.

## Five Element Correspondences

| ELEMENT: | FIRE | EARTH | METAL | WATER | WOOD |
|---|---|---|---|---|---|
| Yin Organ: | Heart/ Pericardium | Spleen | Lungs | Kidneys | Liver |
| Yang Organ: | Small Intestine/ Triple Heater | Stomach | Large Intestine | Urinary Bladder | Gallbladder |
| Tissue: | Blood Vessels | Muscles | Skin | Bone | Tendons |
| Emotion: | Joy | Worry | Grief | Fear | Anger |
| Virtue: | Insight | Empathy | Self-Worth | Courage | Patience |
| Taste: | Bitter | Sweet | Pungent | Salty | Sour |
| Season: | Summer | Late Summer | Autumn | Winter | Spring |
| Climate: | Heat | Dampness | Dryness | Cold | Wind |
| Odor: | Scorched | Fragrant | Rotten | Putrid | Rancid |
| Sound: | Laughing | Singing | Crying | Groaning | Shouting |
| Color | Red | Yellow | White | Dark Blue | Green |
| Sense Organ: | Tongue | Mouth | Nose | Ears | Eyes |
| Movement: | Expanding | Stabilizing | Contracting | Conserving | Generating |
| Function: | Growth | Transformation | Harvest | Storage | Birth |
| Quality: | Enthusiasm | Contentment | Inspiration | Willpower | Creativity |

Each of the elements is associated with different organ systems, colors, tastes, seasons. These correspondences are used in diagnosis and treatment.

Each of the five elements interacts with each of the others in specific ways. The five elements are perhaps more accurately known as the five phases (*wu xing*), reflecting their dynamic, moving nature.

The five elements have both generating and controlling qualities amongst themselves as they interact. In a patient with Lung (metal) ailments—chronic bronchitis or asthma—there is frequently a weak Spleen (earth generates metal). Treatment includes strengthening the Spleen to heal the Lungs.

These are metaphors that help us diagnose and treat imbalances. They do not denote specific organic substances or physiological processes, although we may find correlations to these as research advances.

## Acupuncture Anatomy and Physiology

In Western anatomy, each of the organs has a precise location and distinct set of functions: heart, stomach, liver, kidneys, lungs, gallbladder, and so on. In Chinese medicine, the "organs," while related to anatomy, emphasize functional relationships, and are not equivalent to organs as we know them. The two treatment systems use the same words to mean very different things. In acupuncture, the "Heart" includes the mind, the "Kidneys" include aspects of the endocrine system, and the "Spleen" incorporates parts of the endocrine, immune, and digestive systems, including the pancreas.

Anatomy in acupuncture is defined mainly by the network of meridians that connects the body head-to-toe, and inside to outside. This includes the location of acupuncture points along these meridians, and their connections to the internal organ systems.

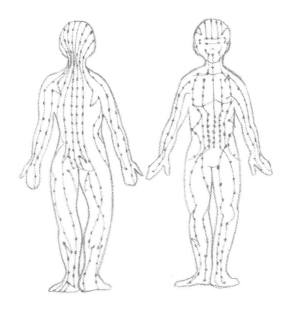

Acupuncture points are found along the meridians that connect all
parts of the body. Stimulating a point on one part of a meridian
sends signals to other areas that it reaches. Through the meridians,
the head can be treated using a point on the foot, and the internal
organs can be treated using points on the arms or legs.

## The Four Vital Substances: Qi, Jin Ye (Fluids), Blood, and Jing (Essence)

Acupuncture refers to four vital substances in the body. They include
*qi*; *jin ye* (body fluids); Blood; and *jing*, essence.

### Qi: Vital Energy

*Qi*, widely translated as "vital energy," is seen as enlivening the whole
body and moving through the meridians. It has sometimes been translated
simply as "vapors" or "breath." Much has been written about its origins
and intended meaning, often drawing on what is signified by its original
Chinese character depicting vapors rising from food.[2]

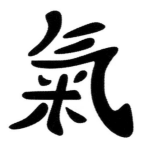

The Chinese character for *qi* depicts vapors rising from food.

In Chinese medicine, the quantity and quality of *qi* in the body and in specific organ systems can be measured, and then manipulated through acupuncture. Does *qi* exist? Is it real or imaginary? If it does exist, does it have an equivalent in Western physiology? We don't know.

Critics scoff at the concept of *qi* flowing through what they consider to be imaginary meridians, and use this to try to debunk acupuncture and shut down the scientific inquiry. A more scientific view takes into consideration that these are two different paradigms and ways of seeing the body. It is unlikely that we will discover some previously unknown substance that is *qi* flowing through the body. Scientifically, *qi* is more likely to represent a combination of biochemical, electromagnetic, and physiological processes that work together to keep the body healthy and alive.

Ancient Chinese healers made observations, and then gave names to what they saw. *Qi* is how they described one form of vitality. Understanding *qi* as something essential to life and health, they developed treatment methods to increase it when it was deficient, to unblock it when it was "stuck," and to redistribute it when imbalanced.

### Jin Ye: Body Fluids

Body fluids—known as *jin ye*—include tears, saliva, sweat, breast milk, and all the fluids that are found in the body. *Jin ye* can be further divided into clearer, lighter fluids that soften and moisten tissues, and thicker fluids involved with the brain, joints, and other parts of the body.

## *Blood*

Blood, also a body fluid, is important enough to be seen as its own form of vital substance. Blood is considered to be essential for the formation of all the tissues and organs, and for keeping the body sufficiently moistened and nourished. Blood and *qi* are closely interrelated. They flow together, and *qi* is considered to be the "commander" of Blood.

In circulation, Blood is the substance that flows while *qi* is the motive force or movement itself. Without *qi*, the Blood doesn't move. Blockage of *qi* will eventually lead to blockage of Blood, a more serious condition in which actual masses can form. Similarly, a loss of Blood will lead to a deficiency of *qi*, which not only propels but travels with the Blood.

## *Jing: Essence*

*Jing*, another vital substance, is known as "essence" and it is the substance that regulates reproduction, growth and development. *Jing*, along with *qi*, is understood to form the foundation for our spirit, known as *shen*. *Jing* is inherited from our parents, so in this sense it includes our genetic constitution as well as reflecting the health of our parents at the time of conception, and the health of our mothers during pregnancy.

Here is a good example of a "non-scientific" Chinese concept now finding support through Western science. Recent studies in the field of epigenetics are revealing how parents' life experiences, and even those of earlier ancestors, can affect a child's health. Ancient Chinese medicine recognized this long before Western science did. Although they expressed it in terms that may sound primitive to us today, this concept has been part of acupuncture practice for thousands of years.

Each of these vital substances is measurable in acupuncture, and each has diagnostic signs and methods of treatment. Yet, none has a precise correlate in Western anatomy and physiology that we know of so far. Even Blood, while it has many properties in common with the substance blood as we know it, has its own unique identity in Chinese medicine and cannot be understood to represent an exact equivalent.

## Acupuncture Diagnosis—The Four Examinations

Ancient Chinese acupuncturists didn't have functional MRIs or blood tests to diagnose a patient, or to measure the effects of their treatment; they used their own senses. The "four examinations" in acupuncture include **looking, feeling, listening** and **asking**.

### *Looking*

An acupuncturist observes the patient's body, including its shape, tone (firm or soft), movement, skin coloration, as well as the appearance of the tongue. Is the face red? Pale? Does it have a greenish hue? Each of these points to different imbalances in the body. What about the eyes? Are they shining and clear, or dull and clouded? Are they red, indicating heat?

The tongue also provides information about imbalances in the body. The acupuncturist observes the color, moisture, coating, as well as any lines or indentations found on the tongue. In the simplest terms, if the tongue is red there is heat; if purplish, Blood stagnation; if it's swollen or has a thick coating, dampness. Different parts of the tongue reflect the health of various organ systems. For example, if there's redness on the sides of the tongue, there is heat in the Liver; a red tip may indicate heat in the Lungs or the Heart.

### *Feeling*

In acupuncture, the pulse is felt on both wrists, in three different positions, at three different depths. Just as regions of the tongue reflect different parts of the body, pulse locations on the wrist also correspond to different organ systems.

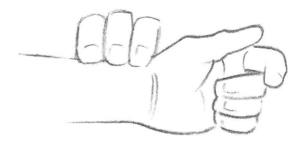

An acupuncturist feels the pulse at three locations on both wrists, and at three depths of pressure. Each position relates to a different organ system: Lungs, Liver, Kidney, Heart, Stomach and so on. The rate is only one of many qualities that are felt to determine the inner workings of the body.

In Western medicine, the pulse is used to determine the heart rate: beats per minute are counted. In Chinese pulse diagnosis, the rate is just one of many qualities that are assessed. We feel for whether the pulse feels "tight" like a wire, "ropy," "soggy," "soft," "floating" (pushing up at a higher level than expected), or "deep" (found only with increased pressure). Other qualities include "slippery," "choppy," "intermittent," and "knotted." A slippery pulse may indicate phlegm in the body; a deep pulse indicates weakness or blockage; a floating pulse may indicate acute infection. Each pulse position relates to a different organ system in the body. Even in the same patient, each pulse location can have its own distinct set of qualities. It can be floating in the first position, slippery in the second, and deep in the third. Putting all this together gives the acupuncturist a good idea of the patient's imbalances, and what treatment is needed.

Pulse reading is used to diagnose the body's imbalances, and to assess treatment responses and recovery. When needles are placed in the selected acupuncture points, the radial pulse qualities change immediately, reflecting a change in the body's internal functions, which in turn leads to healing. For example, if we find a weak, soggy pulse on the Spleen position, corresponding to poor digestion and fatigue, strength returning to that pulse is the first indication that function has improved in the Spleen, leading to improved digestion and reduced fatigue. If we see no change in the pulse after needle placement, the treatment may be modified until the desired change is felt.

In some traditions the abdomen, also known as the *hara* or *dantian*, is palpated, to detect tension, weakness, heat or cold, all of which point to specific meridians or other imbalances in the body.

The meridians may be palpated along the arms and legs, as are specific acupuncture points, to feel for areas of excessive tension, softness, sensitivity or nodules. These findings become part of the diagnosis that leads to a treatment plan for the patient's recovery.

### Listening

"Listening" includes paying attention to both sounds and smells. The sound of the voice may carry tonal qualities associated with the five element correspondences: singing, crying, groaning, shouting, or laughing. To the trained ear of the acupuncturist, these qualities become apparent, and they help provide understanding about the patient's constitution as well as the state of health. Is the voice weak or strong? Quiet or loud? Does it have a singing, shouting or growling quality? Each of these qualities means something in diagnosis.

There may be other sounds such as gurgling in the abdomen or rattling in the chest, all of which give us more information about what is going on in the patient's body. There may be subtle or pronounced body odors that serve as additional diagnostic indicators, again following the five element correspondences, relating to different constitutional types or imbalances. The five element odors are fragrant, rotten, putrid, rancid, and scorched. These tend to be quite subtle and perceptible only to those who are trained to identify them, so you don't have to worry whether your odor is noticeable to others. There are cases where it might be, but in general, it isn't.

### *Asking: The Patient's Story*

Most acupuncturists provide you with an intake form that asks a lot of questions about your health history and symptoms. These will include questions about your health in childhood, and many "little" symptoms that you wouldn't even consider noteworthy, but which mean something in acupuncture diagnosis.

Your story is part of the diagnosis. What is going on? How long has it lasted? What was happening in your life at the time the symptoms started? Do you tend to feel hot or cold? Prefer warm or cold drinks? How is your sleep? Do you fall asleep easily? Once asleep, do you stay asleep or wake up? If you tend to wake up at night, at what time?

A lot of patients feel they're basically pretty healthy "except for the back pain" (or headaches, or whatever symptom they've come in to treat). But once they fill out the intake form, they realize there's a lot more going on that can benefit from acupuncture treatment. If you've had excess weight gain and you also have sugar cravings, that can be treated with acupuncture. It's part of your acupuncture diagnosis and helps in understanding your individual patterns of imbalance, which leads to the most effective treatment. Many symptoms that you've been taking for granted as part of life can actually be treated and eliminated using acupuncture.

# Metaphor in Practice: How it Works

How is metaphor used in acupuncture diagnosis and treatment? Let's take an example: a patient suffering from digestive distress, bloating, cramping, and loose stools. In the language of metaphor, this condition might be seen as "wood attacking earth," also known as "Liver overacting on the Spleen." Treatment would involve using acupuncture points and methods to "sedate" (calm) the Liver, and "fortify" (strengthen) the Spleen. Many of those acupuncture points would be located on the arms and legs—nowhere near the digestive organs—as these are considered among the more potent acupuncture points on the body. "Local" points, on the torso and closer to the digestive system, might be added to support the treatment. The patient would experience a relief of pain, bloating, and diarrhea. The entire treatment would have taken place using metaphor as the guide.

The use of metaphor in acupuncture is often criticized by skeptics. They argue that metaphor is imprecise at best, and inaccurate at worst. This is what I struggled with mightily as a young scientist first studying acupuncture. Everyone knows that an "evil wind" doesn't enter at the back of the neck, causing you to catch a cold, right? On the other hand, how many of us have experienced catching a cold just after being exposed to a chilly draft on the back of the neck—stuck out in the cold rain or sitting under an air conditioner at work?

Our relationship with climate, and its effect on health and illness, matters in acupuncture. This may at first seem primitive or just plain wrong. But those with achy joints know that their joints ache more when rain is coming. Some say that during a humid summer they feel lethargic. Some overheat in summer while others simply cannot get warm in winter. Some find wind intolerable, while for others it's invigorating. When you look at individual responses to weather patterns, you will readily find a related pattern of imbalance in the body.

Over the years, I have come to understand the functional brilliance of the metaphors used in acupuncture. "Liver wind," for example, can lead to twitches and spasms. Western science calls this implausible: there is no "wind" in the liver, and we know that spasms involve the nervous system and muscles. However, this language contains meaning to those who speak it: "wind" is a moving force, and twitches move like wind. More importantly, the diagnosis of "Liver wind" directs the acupuncturist to the appropriate form of treatment. When the correct points are used, the symptoms go away. There's an internal integrity to the medicine: diagnosis leads to treatment leads to cure.

I also find that the use of metaphor frequently helps patients understand what is going on in their own body even better than scientific explanations. This, in turn, helps them understand what they need to do to recover. It helps make sense of myriad symptoms the patient is experiencing, which seem to be random, but are actually all connected. The patient who comes in saying, "I'm a wreck. Everything is falling apart," is a good case in point. This patient has usually been to countless doctors, received numerous scans, tests, and possible disease diagnoses without feeling better. They are scared, confused, and naturally upset, because it seems like energy, well-being and happiness will elude them forevermore.

## Western Medicine or Acupuncture?: Kerry's Story

Kerry came for acupuncture in desperation as a last hope after being to many doctors for her anxiety, sensitive stomach with a sour taste, vertigo, shortness of breath, and pain in her chest, back, side and stomach. She'd been scanned inside and out and given several prescription medications and diagnoses, but felt no better. She was so deeply fatigued that she could barely walk anywhere without becoming exhausted.

*She'd been scanned inside and out and given several prescription medications and diagnoses, but felt no better. She was so deeply fatigued that she could barely walk anywhere without becoming exhausted.*

Kerry had a history of disc problems in her back, and when she was younger she'd occasionally suffered from acid reflux, which would respond to antacids when she needed them. When I met her, she was 54 and menopausal, but the hot flashes she'd had a few years earlier were now gone.

When I heard Kerry's story I learned that she'd been under intense physical and emotional stress for the past two years with a series of crises amongst her family and friends that she'd been managing. During this time she'd also had a bad dental procedure that caused intense nerve pain for one entire year, until another dentist corrected the problem. During that time she'd taken a lot of anti-inflammatory medications (NSAIDs) for the pain. In the last 3-1/2 months her anxiety had become extreme, and the stomach pain and sour taste had started.

Her doctors gave her Valium for the anxiety and Meclizine for her vertigo, which was worse in the mornings and at high altitudes (even though they didn't know what was causing it). She was on statins for high cholesterol, and took occasional laxatives for constipation. She also self-administered some herbs and vitamins which she'd read could help with stomach pain.

Through her CT scans, endoscopy and blood tests, her doctors had determined that she had inflammation of the lower stomach (frequently caused by NSAIDs), no ulcer, no acid reflux, no damage to the esophagus, no tumors, no blood clots, no lung or heart problems, and no H. Pylori infection in the stomach.

What she did have was something resembling achalasia, a condition of unknown origin in which the upper stomach sphincter does not relax to let food in from the esophagus. Her doctors emphasized that though it was similar to achalasia because of the sphincter tension, she didn't have the full profile of that condition, which is associated with other features that she did not have. They advised her to eat small amounts at a time.

Kerry's body signs indicated that her adrenals were exhausted, her digestive system was weak, and all her organ systems were tired. In acupuncture terms she suffered from *qi* and yang deficiency in multiple systems, as well as yin deficiency and *qi* constraint. When the adrenals get exhausted, all the other systems suffer as well and none of the body systems can function optimally, nor can they coordinate with one another as they should. Kerry's heavy use of NSAIDs for dental pain had most likely created the stomach inflammation, adding to her digestive sensitivity and further taxing her adrenals.

Kerry had an extremely tight diaphragm, the muscle that separates the chest from the abdominal cavity. She also had tight muscles over the abdomen, around the side of the body, and in the back. The muscle tension patterns replicated the areas of pain that she had colored in on the human figure in her intake form. She also had very tight muscles in the neck as well as chronic low-level sinus congestion.

*When the adrenals get exhausted, all the other systems suffer as well and none of the body systems can function optimally, nor can they coordinate with one another as they should.*

Adrenal fatigue occurs over time when we live under stress and put out more energy than we're taking in on a daily basis. It's the job of the adrenals to respond to this stress, and they try their best, but finally they just run out of juice. Going through menopause often exacerbates adrenal depletion in a woman. After many years of a demanding career, then menopause, then two years of family crises and one year of dental pain, Kerry's body just collapsed.

At that point, she had no strength to replenish her own body's reserves or to maintain the tone of her musculature. Areas in her body that may have already been a bit tense went into full-blown spasm, including the diaphragm and other muscles around the stomach, side, back and neck. Her immune and digestive systems were both weak, resulting in a chronic irritation of the sinuses, along with congestion.

Combined with her neck tension and low blood pressure, the sinus congestion created vertigo. This was probably a perfect storm of muscles, congested lymphatic fluid and inflammation resulting in pressure on the nerves that are responsible for balance, along with a lack of adequate blood supply. It was worse in the mornings because her head got stuffier from lying down all night, and worse at high altitudes because there was just less oxygen.

Because Kerry's diaphragm was so tense, she couldn't take a deep breath in, and if she tried, she became dizzy. The diaphragm has to contract and relax with each breath in and out. Hers was all locked up and unable to allow this movement.

The doctors had checked her lungs and heart and evaluated her for blood clots to rule out serious causes behind her shortness of breath. But the real reason she was short of breath was that the diaphragm didn't move, and several other muscles in the chest wall were also in chronic spasm, limiting her respiration.

The esophagus passes through the diaphragm on its way to the stomach. With a diaphragm as tight as Kerry's was, it is no wonder that her esophagus couldn't produce muscular waves of contraction to move food into the stomach, or that her sphincter was too tight. All the muscles and tissues in that region were in a stranglehold. It doesn't really matter what caused what in which order – essentially, all the muscles needed to be treated so that they could relax. This would take the iron grip off the region and once again allow proper nerve stimulation to the muscles and blood flow to nourish the organs. How can the stomach digest food or even produce the necessary enzymes when it's being squeezed like that?

Kerry's anxiety was understandable in a body with adrenal and multi-system exhaustion, as well as tightness in the chest and diaphragm. It was as much a physical symptom as an emotional one.

Kerry was given acupuncture to restore her adrenals, her digestion, and to relieve tension and constraint throughout her body so that all the parts could work again.

After her initial treatment she felt more relaxed and less fatigued than she had in a long time. Her diaphragm loosened up and she could take a deep breath without becoming dizzy. The stomach relaxed. She noticed in the next few days that her body temperature, which had been running below 97 degrees (normal is 98.6), had increased by a full degree, and she felt warmer, along with having more energy, less anxiety and a much better mood.

> *Kerry's anxiety was understandable in a body with adrenal and multi-system exhaustion, as well as tightness in the chest and diaphragm. It was as much a physical symptom as an emotional one.*

But Kerry also noticed that small things like a phone call from a friend or agitating news made her side seize up in pain and her sour taste return. With no adrenal reserve and a body so severely depleted, she had no ability to tolerate stress. Every little thing tripped the switch and pushed her into symptoms. Because the muscles weren't fully released, they could easily be pulled back into the pattern of tension. Any remaining spots of tension served as a kind of "stitch in the fabric" that pulled on the other muscles when they got triggered.

Coming back from adrenal exhaustion is like this – it's a jagged recovery with ups and downs. This is because you can't stop living, and life still has stress. Yet, you have no resilience to respond to stress. So it's two steps forward and one step back as you heal.

I advised Kerry to rest as much as possible, to lighten her schedule, and to let her friends and family know she needed their support for her healing. This way she would no longer be the first person to call when they had a crisis. Meanwhile, she came for acupuncture twice a week to restore her body's systems and relieve the patterns of muscle tension.

The medical tests and scans had helped to rule out serious problems, so that Kerry and I could work together with confidence, knowing that there wasn't anything medically critical going on. But that's the only purpose those tests had served for her. None of the treatments that had come from the doctors did anything to help heal her or make her feel better.

Seeing Kerry's body as a whole, looking at the big picture in terms of her history and how it all fits together, it was actually very simple to tell what was going on for her – and how to fix it using acupuncture. Acupuncture restored her energy, her adrenals, her organ functions, and relieved her muscle tension, thereby restoring healthy digestive function and relieving anxiety.

## A Symptom is Not a Diagnosis

The same symptom may have various different causes in different patients, so the symptom is not a diagnosis. It's a label. Let's say you've been given a Western diagnosis such as acid reflux, insomnia or high blood pressure. Then you consult an acupuncturist. The acupuncturist looks for what unique imbalances in your body have created this symptom. Your Western medical diagnosis gives a name to your symptoms or syndrome. Your acupuncture diagnosis identifies patterns of imbalance that underlie your symptoms. The goal, symptom relief, is accomplished by resolving your unique imbalances and not by suppressing the symptom itself.

For example, let's take insomnia. In acupuncture, one sleepless patient might have a pattern of deficient Liver Blood. Another patient might have Spleen *qi* deficiency causing insufficient Heart Blood, also causing insomnia. Each of these patients would exhibit different types of insomnia: one may have trouble falling asleep and another can fall asleep but has difficulty staying asleep. Another patient may have constrained Liver *qi* – causing an awakening at 2 a.m. like clockwork – and someone else may have blocked flow between the Liver and Lung meridians – waking that patient at 3 a.m. Each of these patterns would be treated differently with acupuncture.

> *Your Western medical diagnosis gives a name to your symptoms or syndrome. Your acupuncture diagnosis identifies patterns of imbalance that underlie your symptoms. The goal, symptom relief, is accomplished by resolving your unique imbalances and not by suppressing the symptom itself.*

The insomnia patient with Liver Blood deficiency will often show completely normal lab results on standard blood tests. This means that the acupuncture diagnosis of Blood deficiency doesn't necessarily translate into anemia or any other clinically measurable blood problem. In addition to insomnia, this patient will often suffer from depression, dizziness, and the appearance of floaters in the field of vision. The Western physician will typically prescribe an SSRI antidepressant, such as Prozac, and a sleep aid such as Ambien to control the two major symptoms, but will not address the dizziness and floaters; nor has the underlying condition been resolved.

In the same patient, there are acupuncture points to treat the pattern of Liver Blood deficiency. Using these points will resolve all the symptoms: depression, insomnia, dizziness, and floaters. So in this respect, the "diagnosis" of Liver Blood deficiency is arguably more accurate than the Western diagnosis, which focuses only on the symptoms. In Western science we don't yet know what comprises "Liver Blood deficiency" physiologically, nor do we have a method for treating its root.

# Paths to Healing: Acupuncture's Many Approaches

An acupuncturist treats a patient using various models: yin and yang, five elements, and points both on and off meridians. Multiple – and even contradictory – systems are well tolerated in acupuncture practice. Most acupuncturists today will readily shift with some ease to alternative models as needed to achieve clinical results, without negating anything.

You may notice that numerical patterns are frequently encountered in acupuncture's systems of thought and treatment. The number five, for example, is widely used: five elements, five methods of treatment, five transport points. The number of acupuncture points along the body's meridian system is said to be 365. It is not simply a coincidence that this is the precise number of days in the year. It is probably related to the ancient perception of patterns and relationships between humans and nature and a belief in their significance. Perhaps it served at times as a device to assist with memorization within a largely oral tradition of study and learning. The ancient Chinese were drawn to numerical patterns and used them with regularity.

# Acupuncture Styles

Thanks to its long history, acupuncture has many styles associated with different regions and countries. Traditional Chinese Medicine, also known as TCM, is a style of acupuncture that was formulated in the 1950s and 1960s in Mao-era China.[3] Classical acupuncture styles, originating prior to this development, take many different forms, like dialects of language that diverge over the course of time. Rooted in the same theory, each style emphasizes different types of diagnosis and treatment. Each has "favorite" acupuncture points that are used more than others, or slightly different ways of locating the points.

> *Thanks to its long history, acupuncture has many styles associated with different regions and countries.*

Acupuncture needling techniques also vary between styles. Chinese acupuncture tends to use a strong and deep needling approach while Japanese acupuncture uses a lighter, more superficial needling, with finer needles. Trigger point acupuncture uses a pecking technique in specific locations to relieve pain syndromes. One style of Korean acupuncture focuses on a microsystem of points in the hand to treat the whole body. Likewise, auricular acupuncture, elucidated by Dr. Paul Nogier in France in the 1950s and later adopted by the Chinese, uses the outer ear to treat the entire body. Yet another approach views the abdomen as a microsystem of points to treat the entire body.

## Worsley Five-Element Acupuncture

One of the many acupuncture styles that is widely practiced in the U.S. is a distinct approach taught by Professor J.R. Worsley. This style of acupuncture is infused with more spiritual or esoteric elements than TCM. One approach is not necessarily more valid or effective than the other—although among acupuncturists this topic is often hotly debated—but there are differences.

In Worsley Five-Element Acupuncture, the acupuncturist identifies the primary underlying elemental imbalance (fire, earth, metal, water, or wood) within the individual, originating at birth or in early childhood. This elemental imbalance, identified through observations made within an extensive interview process, is known as one's "causative factor." The treatment uses acupuncture to balance the patient in relation to it, no matter what symptoms arise. This theory holds that balancing an individual within their own element inherently serves to rectify any imbalances in their system.

By contrast, TCM style acupuncture uses the five elements primarily as diagnostic indicators and guides to treatment. Individuals may also be seen to express one element most strongly, making someone predominantly an "earth" type while someone else might be a "water" type. This tends to lead to ailments typical of that element. For example, a wood type might suffer more from anger and Liver problems, an earth type may gain weight more readily or suffer more fluid retention or allergies, while a fire type might be more prone to anxiety and heart conditions. In TCM, acupuncture is given to treat whatever imbalances are found in the body, regardless of the patient's primary element.

Another distinguishing feature of Worsley Five-Element Acupuncture is its emphasis on "spirit," a part of human wholeness that participates in health and wellness. In treatment, points may be selected based on their ability to treat the patient's spirit. Accordingly, acupuncture points possess names that express their "spirit" and their ability to treat the spirit level in a patient. For example, any acupuncture style sees anger and frustration as a Liver imbalance, yet a Worsley Five-Element acupuncturist might specifically select Acupoint Liver 14, "Gate of Hope," located on the torso, in a patient when frustration or disappointment has led to hopelessness. Acupoint Governing Vessel 12, "Body Pillar," located along the upper spine, is used to restore the central strength that allows a person to hold up under stress and stand up for oneself. Acupoint Triple Heater 5, "Outer Frontier Gate," located on the forearm, may be used to help an individual express outwardly, forming healthy relationships in all arenas of life – friends, family, work – and assisting in creative expression. These are just a few examples of how acupoints can be used to support a person's spirit in this form of acupuncture.

TCM is the core curriculum in most but not all American acupuncture colleges, though it is often supplemented with instruction in alternate styles.

# Acupuncture Styles and Techniques

**Chinese acupuncture** tends to use thicker and longer needles with stronger stimulation.

**Japanese acupuncture** uses finer needles, more superficially inserted.

**Korean acupuncture** is known for using points on the hand to treat the whole body.

**Tuina** (pronounced "twee-na") is a manual therapy often used in combination with acupuncture. It combines massage, acupressure and manipulation of limbs and joints to remove blockages and restore the free flow of qi. It is used for both internal and external disorders, and may utilize application of herbal plasters, liniments, ointments or heat along with manual manipulation.

**Cupping** is the application of glass jars that create suction over areas of muscle tension or internal disease to stimulate blood flow and lymphatic drainage while relaxing connective tissue. It can leave characteristic "marks" of discoloration on the skin that fade on their own, usually within days. Cupping has been traditionally used in many regions of the world beyond China, including Central and Eastern Europe and the Middle East. American patients often recall their parents or grandparents, who came from some of these regions, using cupping on them when they were children as a home remedy for many common ailments including colds, flu and bronchitis.

**Gua Sha** is the application of a stroking technique using a firm object (traditionally a porcelain spoon or a coin; nowadays often a flat stone or metal jar lid is used) to relieve tension or congestion and promote circulation of blood and lymph for healing.

**Moxibustion** is the practice of treating acupuncture points with heat. The herb mugwort, also known as "moxa," has warming properties and is applied over the points to stimulate them. This treatment may be used alone or in combination with acupuncture. It can be applied directly to the skin, held above the surface of the body, or added on top of a needle in variations of direct and indirect moxa therapy.

**TCM** (Traditional Chinese Medicine) was created in Mao-era China in the 1950s-60s and is a variant of ancient Chinese medicine with arguably a more Western medical orientation.

**Worsley Five-Element Acupuncture** often involves inserting needles only briefly, instead of leaving them in place. Taught by Professor J.R. Worsley, this style emphasizes balancing a patient's "causative factor" over treatment of symptoms. This style has a unique system of diagnosis and treatment.

**Auricular acupuncture** is the use of points on the outer ear to treat the whole body. It was developed in Europe and brought to China in the 20th century. It has become known for its use in weight loss and addiction recovery, though it can be used for many more conditions.

**All acupuncture needles** in the United States are required by law to be sterile and disposable, used only once. They are made of stainless steel and are known as filiform needles: needles with no aperture for fluids, in contrast to hypodermic needles used by medical doctors.

## New Approaches to Ancient Techniques

Acupuncture in the West today includes contemporary interpretations of ancient techniques. Because it is a living art, clinical experience informs the present day acupuncturist just as it did the ancient acupuncturists. You will also come across some apparently new treatment approaches. These include newly innovated techniques and elaborations of ancient ones.

The use of electrical stimulation with acupuncture is a more recent application, as are the use of magnets, piezoelectric stimulation devices and "ion-pumping cords" as developed by Dr. Manaka in Japan and introduced to the West by Kiiko Matsumoto, who herself teaches a unique style of Japanese acupuncture.

Among the most widely used "new styles" of acupuncture are auriculotherapy – using points on the ear to balance the whole body – trigger point release, and treatment of motor points. These Western acupuncture treatment styles merit a bit more elaboration.

## Ear Acupuncture: Auriculotherapy

Dr. Paul Nogier (1908-1996) was a French physician who, in the 1950s, developed a system of acupuncture using points on the outer ear, which came to be known as auriculotherapy.[4] Dr. Nogier reportedly received patients in his clinic who each had a scar on a certain point on the upper ear. When he inquired, he was informed that each one of them had been to a local healer who had treated the point with scarring heat for relief of sciatica, and that they had indeed been relieved of their pain.

Dr. Nogier tried this treatment on his own sciatica patients and found that their pain was also relieved. He then experimented with other methods, including acupuncture needles, and found that these worked as well. If this one point on the upper ear was effective in relieving sciatic pain, Dr. Nogier reasoned, there might be other points on the ear to treat other parts of the body. He went on to discover "the man in the ear," also known as the homunculus, a representation of an inverted fetus overlaid onto the outer ear surface, the auricle. Using the image of a fetus as a guide, each organ and every part of the body could be mapped to a specific ear point and used for treatment with acupuncture. While empirical treatment of selected ear points was previously known in China and other parts of the world, Dr. Nogier was the first to find a systematic correspondence between ear points and the whole body.

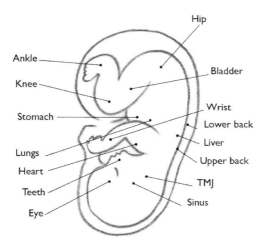

Acupuncture points on the ear can be used to
treat corresponding areas of the body.

The map of acupuncture points on the ear is a microsystem – similar to the reflexology points on the foot – in which the entire body is represented in one of its parts.[5] Other microsystems that have been developed include the hand, face, nose, abdomen, arm and leg. Although there are no direct nerve connections between the ear and the rest of the body, the nerves from the ear are connected to centers in the brain which, when stimulated, send signals through the spinal cord to all parts of the body. Within the microsystem of the ear, functional points have been identified that treat specific conditions, such as hypertension, appetite control, and antihistamine effects.

Dr. Nogier's findings were taken to China in the 1950s and became the subject of intensive research. Through their studies, Chinese researchers verified the clinical effectiveness of the ear points and generated their own map of point locations, remarkably similar to the one created by Dr. Nogier. Ear acupuncture became one of the techniques used by the Barefoot Doctors who were dispatched throughout China as medics during the Cultural Revolution.

Presently in the United States, ear acupuncture is used in conjunction with traditional meridian acupuncture. It can be used on its own or in combination with body points. It has been popularly promoted for use in appetite control and quitting smoking, and there is evidence that it is effective for both.[6] Because of its convenience and ease of application, it has proven to be an effective approach for treatment of soldiers in active duty for pain syndromes, for veterans suffering from post-traumatic stress, and in addiction recovery programs.[7] Sometimes ear points are treated with stick-on magnets or pellets that are worn home to continue stimulating the points for several days in the treatment of pain, for quitting smoking, or for appetite control, weight loss, stress relief, and for relief of nausea in pregnancy.

## Trigger Point Release: Pain Relief and Beyond

Dr. Janet Travell (1901-1997) was a cardiologist and a medical scientist. In addition to her many scientific and medical accomplishments, and no doubt in recognition of these, she served in the 1960s as physician to President Kennedy and subsequently to President Johnson.

As is so often the case when new techniques are innovated, Dr. Travell's interest in musculoskeletal pain patterns began with her own arm pain. By massaging muscles over her shoulder blade in just the right way, she discovered that certain sore spots, when pressed, reproduced the radiating pain she was experiencing down her arm.

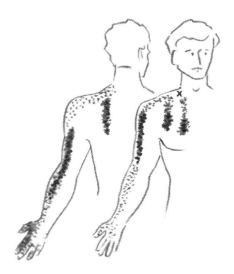

A trigger point in the neck region (x) causes referred pain into the chest and the arm, shown here as shaded areas. Each trigger point in the body is associated with its own characteristic referred pain. Releasing the trigger point relieves the referred pain as well.

As a cardiologist, Dr. Travell came upon studies that reported on persistent pain in the shoulder region following heart attacks, even post-surgery – pain that also radiated down the arm and up the neck on the same side. A series of research projects led by Dr. Travell and spanning several decades identified "trigger points" – spots within the muscle body that were keeping the muscle in spasm.

Dr. Travell observed that trigger points involved not only muscles but also fascial connective tissue, which covers and interpenetrates muscles and all other tissues and structures of the body. This combination of muscle and fascia is known as *myofascia*. Because of the way the body is designed, trigger points tend to show up in specific locations in each muscle group. Dr. Travell mapped the location of trigger points throughout the whole body, including their referred pain patterns.

Dr. Travell also found that organ disease could cause myofascial trigger points in muscles over the organs. Conversely, myofascial trigger points could produce dysfunction in the organs underlying them.[8] Heart patients with persistent arm and shoulder pain were suffering from residual trigger points in the muscle of the chest wall over the heart even after surgery had repaired the heart. When these trigger points were released, the pain went away.

Physiologically this makes sense. When there is a chronic muscle spasm, the blood circulation and innervation in and out of that region will be physically blocked. This results in a build-up of chemicals and metabolic waste products, and an inability for the tissue to receive healthy nutrition and oxygen from the blood, among other things. If this is happening in close proximity to an organ, it stands to reason that this organ will also receive reduced blood circulation, less nutrition and oxygen, impeded nerve supply, and be less capable of clearing away its metabolic waste products. The whole region is "jammed up." The same condition can occur anywhere in the body connected to digestive disorders, upper respiratory problems, and reproductive and fertility issues.

In acupuncture this is axiomatic: where the interior is deficient, the exterior will be relatively excess, and where the exterior is excess, the interior will be relatively deficient. This is another way of saying that heart disease will cause tension in the muscles around the heart over time, and vice versa. Muscle tightness is a form of "excess" because it is strained and blocked. For optimal results, both aspects – internal and external – must be treated together. In acupuncture, we do this by using points to strengthen the internal organs even as we use trigger point needling to release the external tension patterns.

## What is a Trigger Point?

In the course of her research, Dr. Travell described the trigger area in the myofascia as "a link in a self-sustaining cycle of noxious nerve impulses between the central nervous system and the peripheral structures."[9] She found that myofascial tissue, once mechanically stressed through strain, repetitive motion, or injury, or by internal organ disease, can remain in a state of spasm indefinitely. Stimulating the trigger point area with insertion and manipulation of a needle broke the electrical holding pattern and allowed the muscle to return to its normal resting state, relieving the patient's pain.

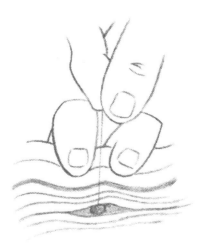

Acupuncture is used to stimulate the trigger point, shown here as a nodule in the muscle body. This induces the trigger point to release in a "twitch response," releasing the spasm and relieving pain by eliminating its source.

Initially, Dr. Travell tried injecting an anesthetic into the trigger point, thinking that this might serve to block the nerve stimulation that was causing the myofascial tissue to remain in spasm. Later she discovered that stimulation by the needle alone served the same purpose. She was able to identify a trigger point by a characteristic "twitch response" elicited when the area was pinched (the muscle "jumps"). The myofascial tissue would twitch under the fingers and that would simultaneously reproduce the referred pain pattern extending into other areas. By needling that location in just the right way, a series of twitch responses could be induced, leading to the relaxation of the myofascial holding pattern and a return of the muscle to its normal state, no longer in chronic spasm.

## Dry Needling

Because she was using the tools she had at hand – hypodermic needles that were ordinarily used for fluid injections – Dr. Travell called this approach "dry needling," as it was done without introducing any fluid. "Dry needling" is therefore the term commonly used by Western health providers – physicians and physical therapists – for this style of acupuncture. It has caused some confusion and more than a little controversy when non-acupuncturists attempt to add this therapy to their scope of practice with minimal training, calling it "dry needling" as though it were not acupuncture. It is acupuncture; however when known as "dry needling" it is a needling technique that is isolated and used outside the context of acupuncture theory.

## New Discovery of an Old Technique?

By her own account, attracted by her reports of "dry needling" on myofascial trigger points to relieve pain, Dr. Travell was visited at Cornell University by acupuncturists from China who had never seen the method she was using. By this time, acupuncture in China was already reformatted from its pre-Maoist styles. These Chinese acupuncturists treated the acupuncture points "by the book" without using palpation to locate tight, tender points; nor did they employ the type of release techniques on muscles that she had discovered. However, Dr. Travell also cites a publication from the early 1900s (pre-Mao) by a Western physician, attesting to the use of acupuncture stimulation in the muscles of the lower back to achieve immediate pain relief. This suggests that an earlier technique may have been lost to Mao-era, TCM style acupuncturists.

My hunch – which I have no way of proving – is that myofascial trigger point release was a form of treatment of so-called "ah-shi" points in earlier forms of acupuncture. Ah-shi points (loosely translated as "yes, there's the point!") are known in acupuncture as points that elicit tenderness upon palpation, whether on or off meridian pathways. On the other hand, Dr. Travell may have discovered this technique for the first time. Either way, we now have a method of myofascial release for pain relief using acupuncture that is highly effective and which elicits immediate and lasting pain relief.

## Find the Pain; Look Elsewhere for the Source

Because of the way pain is referred to regions distant from the spasm or injury, the location of your pain may not be the origin of your pain. The body is a three dimensional structure with interconnecting parts. If the foot is injured it may lead to a limp, which in turn may push the hip into the socket and twist the pelvic bones, and this in turn can alter the position of the shoulders and neck. This patient may come in for treatment of neck and shoulder pain. Because the problem started in the foot and made its way up through the hips and back, the neck will only recover once the lower body is treated, because that's where the source lies.

In any one region there can be multiple active trigger points needing treatment. When treating the shoulder for example, trigger points are likely to be found in several muscle groups, on the front and back of the upper body, as well as the side

> *Because of the way pain is referred to regions distant from the spasm or injury, the location of your pain may not be the origin of your pain.*

and top of the arm, and in the neck – all of which must be treated for full recovery.

In order to relieve pain completely, it's essential for the patient to identify and eliminate any behaviors contributing to the creation of the pain syndrome. For example, many people develop chronic pain in the neck and back due to their sitting posture at the desk or the computer. The posture must be changed or the trigger points will reoccur, along with their characteristic pain syndromes.

## Recent Developments in the Treatment of Trigger Points

Ongoing research has provided an even better scientific understanding of myofascial trigger points. It shows that these areas have an abnormally acidic pH. There's also an increased level of inflammatory and other biochemicals involved in local pain reception. After the trigger point is released through a needle-induced twitch response, levels of these pain-activating substances drop significantly, coinciding with reduced pain and reduced muscle tension. It isn't yet known whether this relief is due to increased blood flow through the area or some other more direct effect on the pain receptor function.[10]

Building upon Dr. Travell's discoveries, trigger point acupuncture has been developed and taught in the West, most notably by Mark Seem, Ph.D., a licensed acupuncturist and educator. Seem has taken the myofascial release work of Dr. Janet Travell and reframed it within the classical acupuncture paradigm, a system he has termed "Acupuncture Physical Medicine."[11] Among his original contributions – again, in a sense, a rediscovery of the ancient practice – he presents a method for treating myofascial holding patterns that includes the whole person and not just the area of pain. In the classical system of Chinese medicine structural imbalances and pain are inextricably connected to the health and physiology of the body as a whole.

## Motor Point Acupuncture

A related approach to myofascial pain relief that has been developed using Western concepts involves treatment of motor points using acupuncture and electrostimulation.[12] Motor points are located where the nerve bundle attaches to the muscle. Many motor points are also known acupuncture points.[13] They are not necessarily the same as trigger points and a different needling technique is used. Yet, motor point acupuncture may also cause a muscle to jump in response to treatment. Motor points are most often used in the area of pain but some have been found – like many acupuncture points – to affect myofascial tissues at some distance away in completely unrelated muscle groups. Motor point acupuncture is frequently presented as a form of sports medicine.

Acupuncture remains an evolving form of medicine. These are but a few of the most prominent innovative forms of acupuncture that are widely used in the West today. As long as acupuncture remains in practice, new styles will continue to emerge, just as new perspectives will emerge as science studies it.

## Key Points

- Acupuncture uses metaphors from nature and society to understand illness.
- Yin and Yang and the Five Elements are the two main metaphorical systems used in acupuncture.
- The four "vital substances" in acupuncture are qi, Blood, jin ye, and jing.
- Shen, the human spirit, arises out of qi and jing.
- The Four Examinations in clinical acupuncture are looking, feeling, listening and asking.
- Diverse acupuncture styles have developed in different parts of the world over time.
- All acupuncture needles in the U.S. are required to be sterile and disposable, used only once.

- Auriculotherapy is the treatment of points on the outer ear using acupuncture.
- The map of acupuncture points on the ear was developed in the 1950s in France by Dr. Paul Nogier.
- Ear acupuncture is an alternative approach to use of meridian points on the body. It can be used on its own or in combination with meridian acupuncture treatment.
- Electro-stimulation of acupuncture points is a 20th century development most often used to enhance acupuncture's pain-relieving effects..
- Acupuncture for release of trigger points was developed by Dr. Janet Travell, who mapped the location of trigger points in muscles throughout the entire body.
- Trigger point release within the system of acupuncture has been further developed by licensed acupuncturist and educator, Mark Seem.
- Trigger point release is widely used for pain relief but is also used in the treatment of internal disorders.
- "Dry needling" is the name given to trigger point release when it is used outside the context of acupuncture theory by non-acupuncturists.
- The source of pain in any area is often found in another part of the body and must be treated for the pain to resolve.
- Motor points, located where nerve bundle attaches to the muscle, are sometimes treated with acupuncture as a form of sports medicine, to relieve pain and improve function.

# CHAPTER THREE

· · · · · · · · · · · · · · · · · · · · ·

# Acupuncture Healing Stories

"It takes a thousand voices to tell a single story"
– Native American saying

I met a healthy, active 80-year-old man who told me that in the previous ten years the health of most of his friends had seriously started to fail, and many had died. They didn't realize that to remain healthy into the 70s, 80s, and beyond, they had to make healthy lifestyle changes in their 30s, 40s, and 50s. Of course there are some things we cannot control about our aging. But it remains true that the way we live now not only affects the quality of our life today, it also sets the stage for how we age.

Those who are struggling with age-related ailments – who have difficulty walking, who are evidently in pain, who are taking several different medications every day – they didn't do anything different from what you – if you're younger – are doing now. This is "normal" aging without healthy intervention earlier on in life. We're all on the same trajectory unless we do something to change it. The reason that diseases of old age are so hard to treat is because they are the result of processes in our bodies that have been progressing for decades. And yet, acupuncture does help relieve pain and other conditions that come with aging.

As changes occur throughout our lives, each stage of growth and maturity has its own set of challenges. Because acupuncture optimizes the body by removing blockages to its own healing abilities, it can be used at every age. It is also a preventive form of treatment. The more balanced you are, the better able you are to ward off illness and injury.

Starting at birth, babies begin taking in nutrition and digesting it for the first time. They grow and develop quickly while being exposed to infections, injuries, and other environmental stress. In addition there can be birth trauma—observed or not—that affects a child's health, development, and behavior, as well as emotional influences from the family, particularly the primary caregivers.

Moving through puberty and into adolescence, children mature physically and emotionally and undergo significant hormonal changes and issues of identity and place in the world while dealing with stresses at home, school and in the community.

Young adults in their 20s have moved from childhood to independence, and for many this involves college, often while working one or more jobs. They proceed into higher education and the job market, starting a career, trying to learn and perform well in new adult environments, all the while learning to be self-supporting, figuring out relationships and sometimes marrying and having children. By the time they reach their mid to late 20s and early 30s, young adults may find themselves burning out in ways they didn't anticipate and don't understand—experiencing anxiety and depression, insomnia, injuries, body pains, and exhaustion.

Throughout their 30s people are typically building their foundation as adults, often starting families and raising children while maintaining challenging careers, and noticing the beginnings of unexpected physical challenges that come with a slightly aging body. Frequently, injuries or illnesses sustained in adolescence begin to reappear as unexplained problems. Old whiplash injuries that seemed to be gone may create painful neck and shoulder pain. Ankle or knee injuries sustained as kids or teenagers produce back and hip pain, or the knees now require surgical intervention. Small problems that once resolved on their own now hang on and get worse. Repetitive strain injuries commonly emerge at this stage— working at the desk and computer, pushing the baby stroller, carrying heavy bags—all things we used to do without any trouble are now causing pain.

By the 40s the body's aging process makes itself more known, and many of us find ourselves more easily injured through activity, exercise, or what we used to consider normal exertion. You fatigue more easily. You might hear yourself saying, "I think I'm just getting old." At this stage more chronic problems begin to set in, including weight gain, the beginnings of high blood pressure and diabetes, arthritis, sciatica, repetitive strain injuries, and disc-related problems in the back and neck.

Women in their 40s often begin to experience hormonal changes associated with perimenopause. This frequently occurs against the backdrop of raising children or teenagers while maintaining a demanding career. I often treat mothers going through perimenopause just as their daughters are hitting puberty, and the hormonal storm of this combination is quite surprising to both. At the same time,

> *By the 40s the body's aging process makes itself more known, and many of us find ourselves more easily injured through activity, exercise, or what we used to consider normal exertion.*

people may be beginning to care for their own aging parents, so while their own physical needs are increasing, so are their levels of responsibility and stress.

During the 50s and 60s, the pressures of later adulthood begin to appear. The body changes in palpable ways that may include chronic illnesses (if maintaining health hasn't been addressed earlier), a noticeable change in energy levels, reduced muscle mass, tone, and strength, insomnia, sexual dysfunction, and new, sometimes complex problems associated with hormonal imbalances and deficiencies.

Many move into their 70s, 80s, and 90s adjusting to an older body in decline. In the best case, we have been caring for our health over the decades and respond quickly and appropriately to problems that arise. Injuries occur more easily and the body is slower to recover. The body needs more attention, proper exercise and rest, and work levels need to be modulated. At this stage many chronic problems become apparent—severe arthritic joint degeneration, spinal stenosis, coronary artery blockage, prostate enlargement or impotence in men, urinary dysfunction in men and women, and so on. It's also the time of onset of other chronic, degenerative diseases, strokes, and loss of hearing and eyesight, including cataracts. A glance at pharmaceutical ads presents a good picture of aging's common ailments.

However, in many cases you don't need to turn to drugs to treat your symptoms. Most of these ailments can be treated using acupuncture and other manual therapies, exercise, rest, and nutrition. By taking this approach you are not only resolving your symptoms, as medications are doing (along with risks of multiple and potentially severe side-effects), but you are improving your health and longevity—without the risks.

## A Word About Stress

To really understand health, illness, and healing, it's important to understand stress and its effects. Stress can be physical, emotional, or environmental. An injury is stress, emotional extremes – anger, sadness, grief – are all forms of stress. Stress doesn't necessarily feel bad. Some of the great celebrations of life are experienced as stress by the body: a promotion, marriage, a new baby. You can be very happy and very stressed at the same time. And of course there are the things we know are stressful: finances, relationships, family responsibilities, tragedies, losses, and deaths. Because stress is inherent in being alive, our bodies are designed to respond to it. However, we're not designed to live in relentlessly high levels of stress as we do today.

> *Because stress is inherent in being alive, our bodies are designed to respond to it. However, we're not designed to live in relentlessly high levels of stress as we do today.*

By design, stress triggers reactions in the nervous system that in turn affect the hormones and every organ in the body. When a threat is perceived, the body goes into survival mode, commonly known as the "fight-or-flight" response. When the cave man encountered a bear, the fight-or-flight response geared his body for maximum strength to either fight it or flee. The heart rate speeds up, the digestion slows down, and breathing accelerates, among many other changes. It's meant to be a short-term reaction. Once the threat has passed, the nervous system normalizes, the heart rate and breathing slow down, digestion functions again, and hormonal balance is restored.

In response to stress, our adrenal glands, located on top of the kidneys, secrete two main hormones: adrenaline and cortisol. Adrenaline increases our heart rate, blood pressure, and helps us access quick energy. Cortisol helps to balance unwanted side-effects of that initial response, fighting inflammation, helping replenish energy reserves, and boosting immune function.

A problem arises when stress becomes perpetual. These days we don't have to fight or run from wild animals, but we push ourselves in ways that simulate that scenario as far as our bodies are concerned. Most of our ailments are directly related to a stress response in overdrive, which eventually weakens us and leads to multi-system breakdown.

In the initial stage of chronic stress, we're secreting too much cortisol and our blood levels are elevated. This leads to elevated blood sugar levels, which in turn stimulates increased insulin secretion by the pancreas. If left unchecked, this cycle leads to insulin resistance, weight gain, and ultimately, diabetes. The chemical changes associated with chronic stress also lead to high blood pressure, elevated cholesterol, atherosclerosis and heart disease.

In the later stages of chronic stress, we've exhausted our adrenals. Though they are still trying to produce cortisol, they just don't have the reserves to do so. Our blood levels of cortisol are too low. At this point we're exhausted, the digestive system is impaired, the immune system doesn't function properly so we're prone to frequent infections as well as inflammatory conditions of all kinds. We may suffer from insomnia, fatigue, depression, anxiety, sadness, and even hopelessness. Because cortisol uses the same chemical building blocks needed for our reproductive hormones, this stage of chronic stress is associated with abnormally low levels of estrogen, progesterone, and testosterone. This, in turn, affects our sexual and reproductive health as well as cognitive function, energy, metabolism and mood.

Acupuncture works to relieve the effects of chronic stress while restoring the health of the adrenals and all the interconnecting organ systems. In virtually all of the adult

> *Acupuncture works to relieve the effects of chronic stress while restoring the health of the adrenals and all the interconnecting organ systems.*

patient healing stories that follow, chronic stress has played a part in the patient's disease. Acupuncture doesn't speak in terms of the autonomic nervous system, adrenaline and cortisol; it uses terms like Kidney yin and yang deficiency, Kidney and Spleen *qi* deficiency, hyperactivity of Liver yang, and so on, to describe observed imbalances resulting from chronic stress. Acupuncture treatment is aimed at multiple body systems at once to help the patient heal, restore and recover. No such treatment exists in conventional medicine.

## The Healing Stories

Following are stories of patients receiving acupuncture. With each story, I display the patient's age and his or her presenting complaint – the reason they came in for acupuncture. Under that are listed their secondary complaints. These are additional problems that have shown up in the health intake or in the course of examination and treatment. No one has just one symptom or one imbalance. Through these stories, you will see how the whole person is addressed. Individual symptoms that exist in one person are part of one story, one system out of balance in several ways, and they are treated together using acupuncture.

## Acupuncture for Children

Some people are surprised to hear that acupuncture can be used to treat children. "What do you treat them for?" they ask. Children are typically treated for all the common childhood ailments: colds, coughs, asthma, sore throat, teething in babies, colic and other digestive problems, ear infections, pediatric allergies and eczema, bedwetting, as well as sleep problems and certain behavioral or developmental issues.

> ## Conditions Commonly Treated with Acupuncture in Infants and Children
>
> - Colic
> - Constipation
> - Diarrhea
> - Teething
> - Ear Infections
> - Colds and Cough
> - Sore throat
> - Fever
> - Asthma
> - Allergies
> - Eczema
> - Bedwetting
> - Sleep problems
> - Behavioral problems

How well do children tolerate acupuncture? Very well. Most of us got our fear of needles from early experiences having injections at the doctor's office, and we assume that children will be even more averse to the idea of acupuncture than we are. But this is generally not the case. For kids, everything is new, all the time. Acupuncture is another new and fascinating thing for them to learn about, and they take to it quite well.

Children will often ask to help insert or remove the needles, and they remember where the points are located and want to remind me which point I may want to treat next. In adults, needles are inserted and kept in place for some time, typically twenty minutes or longer, to give the body time to assimilate the changes induced by the needles. But in children, who are like little green growing shoots, the needles are inserted and immediately withdrawn. Kids are more susceptible to disease than adults but also more quickly and easily return to health. Their bodies are so ready to change and aren't fixed in deeper "holding patterns" of imbalance, so this quick stimulation is sufficient; fortunately—because it would be hard for small children to lie still for twenty minutes with needles in place.

How are children treated using acupuncture? A parent may hold the child in his or her lap while the treatment is administered. Depending on their age, many children become comfortable sitting or lying on the treatment table on their own. In addition to acupuncture, it's also possible to treat points with acupressure instead of needles – or with moxibustion, using warming herbs on the points, or with different forms of massage. The Japanese developed little tools and a treatment method for children known as *shonishin*, in which points and meridians are stimulated on the surface of the skin but never punctured.

Herbal medicine can also be used for children. To administer herbs to nursing infants it's even possible to give the herbal formula to the mother, who then passes it on to the baby through her breast milk.

## How Are Children Treated with Chinese Medicine?

A range of approaches may be used or combined in the treatment of children:

- Acupuncture
- Acupressure (using finger pressure on acupoints)
- Shonishin (acupoint stimulation over the skin)
- Massage
- Gua Sha (a specialized form of massage using a hand-held tool)
- Moxibustion (using warming herbs over or on acupoints)
- Dietary changes (can be central to healing in children)
- Herbal medicine formulas – applied to the skin or taken internally

## Healthy Digestion is the Key to a Child's Health

A child's digestive system is immature before the age of six. Therefore, when treating children for almost any ailment, the first line of inquiry, and most influential place to start, is the diet.

In Chinese Medicine, the Spleen and Stomach are the organ systems primarily responsible for digestion. The Spleen's role includes sending *qi* up to the Lungs and Blood to the Heart for distribution through the entire body.

Due to its immaturity in babies and children, the Spleen's function is easily impaired and this in turn starts a chain reaction leading to heat, dampness, phlegm and toxins, or some combination of these factors, which underlie many of the ailments of childhood, including asthma, eczema, ear infections, recurrent sore throats and fevers. Phlegm, while it shows up in the Lungs, originates in a Spleen that is weak, overburdened, and unable to digest foods and transport fluids properly.

Because of their immature digestion, children easily react badly to foods that they can't digest properly, foods that further weaken the Spleen, or overfeeding. This is often complicated and made worse by the repeated use of antibiotics to treat ear and upper respiratory infections in children. It's a vicious cycle in which diet leads to impaired Spleen function, which in turn generates heat and phlegm, leading to ear, lung and throat infections. The use of antibiotics further weakens the Spleen, perpetuating the cycle of infection, which is then followed by more antibiotic use.

Antibiotics are sometimes necessary but are commonly overprescribed. Designed to fight bacterial infections, they also wipe out healthy bacteria in the digestive tract, leading to overgrowth of yeast and fungus. These organisms trigger the immune system, which tries to fight them, and this overworks and weakens it. They can also create an opportunity for undigested food particles to move through the intestinal wall into the bloodstream, a condition known as "leaky gut syndrome." When this happens, the immune system sees these undigested food particles as foreign bodies and attacks them, and this leads to allergic reactions to foods that would otherwise be well-tolerated. This is one cause for common allergic conditions in children, including asthma and eczema.

## Birth Trauma

Birth trauma is almost completely unacknowledged unless it is severe, but it frequently occurs even in the most "normal" of birthing situations, where there is compression to the head or twisting of the body. It can establish patterns in an infant's body that lead to problems later, including developmental and behavioral disorders as well as emotional and structural problems. There may also have been incidents, including stress or illness, in the mother's life during pregnancy that can affect the child later.

## Genetic and Hereditary Issues

There are of course genetic and hereditary issues in children, some of which can be mitigated using acupuncture, and many of which may require multidisciplinary treatment approaches, including conventional medicine, acupuncture, manual therapy, and psychotherapy.

## Family and Home Environment

Finally, a child's home and social environment is frequently involved in his or her ailments, from physical conditions like insomnia, asthma, and digestive disorders to emotional or behavioral problems. When treating the health of a child using acupuncture, the child's complete history and environment, including the health of the parents and home environment, need to be taken into consideration.

## Diagnosing Children

The same principles are used in diagnosing children as in adults. Using the four examinations: looking, listening, feeling and asking, we seek to determine what imbalances are causing symptoms.

Looking involves observation of the child including color of the face, hands, nails, liveliness or "spirit," appearance of the tongue (when possible), mouth, ears, eyes, skin, and the body as a whole. In babies and toddlers there is a vein at the base of the index finger which can be observed for its color, depth, thickness and how far along the finger it extends. Each of these qualities are indicators of patterns of imbalance within the child's body – whether there is heat or cold and how severe the illness might be.

Listening includes paying attention to any sounds including the voice quality and strength, breathing – including wheezing, cough – whether dry, wet or rattling – and noting the quality of any odors, including the child's breath.

Feeling involves touching the child, noting body temperatures and areas of heat or cold, and the quality of muscles as well as the abdomen – whether too soft or too firm. As the child grows it becomes possible to feel the rate and qualities of the radial pulses (on the wrist) for more information about internal disease patterns.

Asking the parents questions about the child's symptoms fills out the diagnosis. When did the problem start? Is there any fever? How does the child sleep? How is the energy level, appetite, mood? I want to know about the child's diet and eating patterns, and about elimination – the quality and odor of urine and stools. It may also be pertinent to explore any birth-related issues such as prematurity or difficult labor and birth, as well as questions about the home and family environment.

## How to Use Acupuncture in the Treatment of Children

When I see children for acupuncture treatment, invariably they are suffering in some way when they come in – typically fever, asthma, cough, ear infection, colic or some other digestive problem. Because their bodies respond so rapidly, you can usually see changes happening right before your eyes as they receive treatment. Depending on the ailment, parents frequently observe rapid recovery within 24 hours after treatment. We may do a series of treatments to bring the child's health back into balance, all the while making necessary dietary changes and sometimes using herbal medicine at the same time.

After recovery, parents learn to bring their children back in for treatment right away when illness arises, before it has a chance to develop. I also teach them home treatment approaches using diet, massage, and other techniques to use to keep the child healthy and to restore balance when the child begins to show signs of sickness. For children, as with adults, using acupuncture for preventive health maintenance is a way to optimize wellness and avert illness.

It's essential for children to have a pediatrician and to receive appropriate medical care as required. Diet, acupuncture, herbs, massage and home treatment can be the first line of defense for most common illnesses. Monitoring by the pediatrician ensures that you will know when your child needs medical treatment. For more severe problems or infections, or if the condition worsens instead of improving, conventional medical treatment is absolutely necessary.

## Dietary Guidelines for Children's Health

Because digestion is not fully mature in children, it's the source of most common childhood illnesses – as well as the key to recovery. Here are some guidelines to help you understand how your child's diet can best support health, starting from birth.

- Whether breastfeeding or not, it's recommended that you feed your infant on a schedule. Feeding on demand often causes overfeeding which leads to food stagnation, heat, and phlegm, predisposing the baby to indigestion, colic, sleep disturbances, ear infections and so on.
- In all children, it's best to eat small quantities more frequently during the day instead of larger, less frequent meals. This is easier on the immature digestive system and keeps it from becoming overburdened and thereby weakened.
- When introducing foods to the diet, start with a single food and see how the child responds. Wait a week before introducing another new food. If there is any unwanted reaction from the food, remove it from the diet immediately. Wait some time before trying it again.
- Feed your young child food that is warm and cooked. Cold and raw foods – including raw fresh vegetables and fruits – are harder for an immature digestive system to handle and can impair the digestive function, creating illness.

- Avoid feeding your child sweet and cold foods, including fruit juice and ice cream. Sweets in general damage the Spleen, and when cold they're even worse.
- Other foods to limit include breads, cheese, nuts (including peanut butter). All of these foods are hard to digest and tend to generate dampness and phlegm, factors underlying most childhood illnesses.

## Zachary: Colic and Insomnia, 7 months

Zachary was suffering from colic and he would cry and fuss for a couple of hours after each feeding. He also woke up regularly at night, crying and screaming. He was breastfed until about four months of age, and then began eating most of the same foods as the rest of the family at meals. There had been no gradual introduction of foods and his young digestive system couldn't handle all that he was being given to eat. As a result, it was generating internal heat and dampness, a pattern that led to colicky pain and insomnia. His mother said that he had a huge appetite and always wanted more food. This is characteristic of heat in the digestive system.

Zachary received acupuncture once a week for six weeks. I advised his mother to change his diet back to very simple foods, focusing on milk and rice at first, and introducing new foods very slowly over the following year. For the first few days, Zachary continued to fuss because he still had an appetite from the heat in the stomach and seemed unhappy about the more restricted diet. He began to pass large, foul-smelling stools and had a temporary exacerbation of insomnia as the heat cleared from his body. After six treatments, in conjunction with dietary changes, Zachary's colicky pain cleared up, and he was sleeping well at night.

*Symptoms*: colicky pain, frequent waking and crying at night
*Observations*: red tongue with greasy yellow coating, tight abdomen, agitation
*Illustrative Treatment*[1]: CV12, LI4, ST36, SP6, BL20, dietary changes at home

## Connor - Pediatric Asthma, age 2

Connor had severe childhood asthma when his mother brought him in. As an infant he had also had pediatric eczema. Asthma ran in Connor's family, his mom told me. His grandfather had suffered from both asthma and eczema all his life, as had other members of the family.

On the day I met him, Connor had been to the emergency room the previous night, where he was diagnosed with a viral lung infection. He was given a steroid injection and inhaler to relieve the extreme inflammation and ease his labored breathing. This was a recurring scenario in his young life whenever an infection would trigger Connor's asthma. His mother didn't want to continue giving him steroids, which are hard on the body over time. Yet, unless his condition improved, he would continue to need these emergency steroid treatments.

While the steroids had helped Connor through his respiratory crisis, he was still very sick on the day I saw him. He had a fever and a lot of congestion in the lungs and sinuses. His tongue was red with a redder tip, indicating heat in the body, and in the Lungs especially. The tongue's thick coating also showed the presence of phlegm.

When Connor returned the next day he was feeling much better. Much of the heat had cleared, the fever was gone, his breathing was better, and the congestion was greatly reduced. His mother was so happy and relieved. She had resorted to the inhaler only once the previous evening when his breathing became a bit labored. I assured her that this would not interfere with our treatment. Our goal was to work our way to the point where he wouldn't need the steroids anymore. In the meantime, using them for crisis intervention was essential.

Within a week, Connor completely recovered. His mother decided to bring him once or twice weekly for a program of treatment aimed at restoring his health and eliminating the asthma. I spoke with her about the importance of diet in his treatment. Like many parents, she wasn't excited about this, and for the time being she decided to work only with the acupuncture. When he later developed an ear infection, she did some additional reading and became convinced that working with his diet was a necessity. She began to make some changes.

Connor's mom eliminated cow's milk from his diet, as well as gluten. She limited his consumption of citrus fruits, which can lead to phlegm due to their raw, cold, sweet nature, and she gave him water at room temperature instead of chilled. This created a notable improvement in Connor's condition when added to the treatments. He stopped having asthma attacks, and when he caught a cold it resolved more quickly and didn't develop into a lung problem.

Connor continued to receive treatments with varying frequency through the age of 5, sometimes to treat an illness and sometimes to support health when he wasn't sick. He enjoyed his sessions and liked to help remove the needles once in place. He came to know the points that are commonly used in his treatment and tried to guess which ones we were going to use. While he sometimes caught the occasional cold, as all children do, they resolved normally and Connor no longer suffered from asthma.

*Diagnosis*: Viral lung infection, asthma
*Symptoms*: fever, cough, congestion, wheezing and difficulty breathing
*Observations*: red tongue with thick coating, lethargy and agitation
*Illustrative treatment*: LI4, LI11, LU7, K6, ST36, CV12, BL20, BL13, GV14, *gua sha* and dietary changes at home

## Henry: Otitis Media (Chronic Earache and Infections), Age 3

Henry was suffering from recurrent ear infections that were repeatedly treated with antibiotics. This is a very common scenario. Any number of things can set off the initial ear infection in a child, but once the antibiotic use begins, it often sets up a pattern that ensures repeated infection. The antibiotic treatment weakens an already immature digestive system and leads to a buildup of dampness and phlegm. This in turn creates congestion leading to heat, an internal environment prone to repeated infections and inflammation. Henry needed treatment to promote flow of *qi* and Blood surrounding the ear and in the head, along with points to strengthen the Spleen and eliminate dampness and heat. I also added

*Any number of things can set off the initial ear infection in a child, but once the antibiotic use begins, it often sets up a pattern that ensures repeated infection.*

points known to strengthen the immune system, which had been strained by the repeated infections.

Henry received treatments twice a week for three weeks, and then once weekly for another three weeks. I gave Henry's mother dietary recommendations to help reduce the dampness and phlegm in his body. I showed her how to perform *gua sha* on his neck and back, rubbing the area with a firm object to clear heat, promote circulation, and drain phlegm from the ear. Henry's ear infections cleared up quickly and completely in response to this treatment.

*Diagnosis*: Ear infection (Otitis media)
*Symptoms*: Ear pain and pulling, crying, feverish
*Observations*: Redness on and around the ear, slightly red tongue with thick coating
*Illustrative treatment*: TH3, TH17, GB20, GB8, CV12, GV14, ST36, K7, "immune points," *gua sha* and dietary changes at home

## Jake: Allergies and Asthma, Age 6

Jake had suffered from seasonal allergies every spring since he was very young. When he caught cold, it always seemed to lead to asthma attacks, which could be quite severe, requiring a nebulizer and occasional hospitalization.

In children, the treatment of allergies, immunity, and asthma involves strengthening the Spleen while regulating the Liver, Lung and Kidneys. The Spleen is a major key to immunity and freedom from allergies, particularly in children. I used acupuncture along with moxibustion and *gua sha* to strengthen Jake's Spleen and Lungs, support the immune system, and regulate all the other systems in the body. Jake began to have fewer colds, and when he did catch cold, he recovered easily, with less asthma. He received acupuncture up to four times per month for about three months over the winter, and by that spring he enjoyed his first allergy-free season.

*Diagnosis*: Seasonal allergies, asthma
*Symptoms*: Sneezing, coughing, lung and sinus congestion, itchy eyes, wheezing, shortness of breath

*Illustrative treatment*: K7, LU7, LI4, LV3, "Immune points," ST36, BL13, BL20, GV14, moxibustion, *gua sha*

**Cecilia: Eczema, Age 6**

Cecilia had patches of eczema around her elbows and knees – red, dry, itchy skin – and sometimes on her face and chest. Her eczema had started in infancy, probably triggered by the early introduction of foods she wasn't ready to digest. Her mother had since made changes to her diet, eliminating dairy, soy, and gluten, which had helped to some degree, but the eczema persisted. Though her diet had subsequently changed, and she was nearing the age when her digestive system would be more fully mature, there was lingering heat and dampness in her body.

Because Cecilia wasn't sure about trying the needles, I used pressure points instead. She found it very soothing and relaxing, and almost fell asleep while being treated. After one session her eczema cleared up completely and never returned. This particularly rapid recovery is common in children, and because she was eating well and growing to the stage of digestive maturity, Cecilia's body mainly needed help in clearing the lingering heat and dampness in order to heal. Once that was gone, the eczema was gone too.

> *Because Cecilia wasn't sure about trying the needles, I used pressure points instead. She found it very soothing and relaxing, and almost fell asleep while being treated. After one session her eczema cleared up completely and never returned.*

*Diagnosis*: Pediatric eczema
*Symptoms*: Red, dry, itchy patches of skin around elbows and knees
*Illustrative treatment*: LI4, LV3, LI11, LU5, SP6, ST36, GB20, BL13, BL20

**Charlie: Childhood Headaches, Fever, Malaise, and Bedwetting, Age 8**

Charlie, age 8, had suffered from headaches and low-grade fevers for several years. He also suffered from occasional bedwetting, which is usually due to weak Kidneys in Chinese medicine. Medically, no significant problems had been diagnosed, and it appeared that there was nothing to be done until a friend told his mother about acupuncture for kids.

Checking Charlie's pulse, tongue, and meridians showed me that his Kidneys and Spleen were weak, the Liver was not regulated, and he had a stressed immune system. It is common for children to suffer from Spleen imbalances because the immature digestive system is vulnerable. But when a child has weakened Kidneys it is usually due to something inherited or something that occurred in utero or at birth. Sure enough, upon taking his history I learned that Charlie had been born prematurely, requiring several weeks of neonatal intensive care before going home.

Charlie was treated with acupuncture to strengthen the *qi* of the Kidneys and Spleen, and to regulate flow of *qi* through the Liver. He reported that immediately after treatment his headache and fever went away, and he felt much better. He received a series of treatments once or twice a week for several weeks, after which his pulses showed much greater balance and strength, his tongue and meridian signs were improved, the bedwetting ended and he was symptom-free.

*Symptoms*: headache, malaise, low-grade fever, bedwetting
*Observations*: dark circles under eyes, pale tongue
*Illustrative treatment*: K7, ST36, SP9, LV3, LI4, GB20, LU7, BL23, BL20, moxibustion, tuina massage on back, shoulders and neck

## Caleb: Migraine, Anxiety, Age 14

Caleb was 14-years-old when his mother brought him for acupuncture. As an adolescent, he was experiencing symptoms characteristic of this stage of childhood. He suffered from migraine headaches, as well as anxiety and stress at school. Caleb was a good student but struggled to sit down to do homework or to study for tests due to the anxiety it caused.

Checking Caleb's pulses and tongue, I found that his Liver was stressed, creating tension and pain, and he had excess blocked energy in the Heart, reflected in his anxiety. His tongue was pale, with scalloped edges, showing a weakness in the Spleen. He had tight muscles in the neck and upper back. There was physical tension in his diaphragm, which was tight and sensitive to pressure. Apart from this, Caleb seemed fundamentally strong and healthy, as you would expect in a 14-year-old boy.

I treated Caleb to regulate his body's energy and release the tight diaphragm. Even though no acupuncture was done near the diaphragm itself, it immediately relaxed by using points on the arms and legs. The *qi* began to flow freely throughout his body.

A tight diaphragm often traps energy in the Heart, which is accompanied by an overactive and obsessive mind. This reflects acupuncture's view of unity between Heart and mind. Insomnia is another common symptom arising from this pattern. Releasing this blockage relieves the constant over-thinking that creates anxiety.

Caleb visibly relaxed during treatment. We talked about some strategies to manage anxiety over schoolwork. Instead of thinking that sitting down to work meant diving into the full project at hand, he could try coaxing himself into it by starting with just a few minutes of work at a time, and take frequent breaks. Caleb liked the idea and thought it might help him over the hurdle of facing the magnitude of the work all at once, and it did.

I wanted to clear up the tension in Caleb's upper back and neck directly using trigger point release but decided to wait until his second treatment. Because he was young and new to acupuncture, I explained to him that I wanted him to get a feeling for it first, before we began to treat the muscles. While regular acupuncture is usually virtually pain-free, trigger point acupuncture causes the muscles to twitch and spasm as they release their tension. It can be an intense and surprising sensation, though momentary, and I wanted Caleb to experience the calmness he got from acupuncture before beginning this phase of treatment. He understood and agreed.

When I saw him a week later, Caleb happily reported that he'd had only one mild headache, and he'd remained much more relaxed all week and was able to study. He found that once he sat down to work, it was easy to continue, and he had managed his anxiety very effectively. He felt the satisfaction of completing his work and was relieved of the stress that had stemmed from his own procrastination.

On his second visit, in addition to the points used initially, I began to use trigger point acupuncture on his neck and shoulders. I repeated this for several weeks until all his back and neck muscles were relaxed and his anxiety pattern was gone. During this time Caleb suffered not a single migraine headache. He continued to receive acupuncture periodically for balancing, especially during busy times at school and around exam time. He found that it kept him free from migraines and able to study without undue anxiety.

*Symptoms*: Recurring migraine headaches, intense anxiety, unquiet mind
*Observations*: Tight diaphragm, pale tongue, tight muscles, constrained Heart and Liver *qi*, weak Spleen
*Illustrative treatment*: LV3, PC6, TH5, GB41, SP9, K4, LI11, GB20, Yintang, Trigger points: upper trapezius, levator scapula, supraspinatus, rhomboids

## Acupuncture for Women's Health

In treating women over the years, I've seen that women's health is generally not met with sufficient information or attention. A woman goes through dramatic hormonal and life changes starting with puberty, moving through to fertility, pregnancy, childbearing, mothering, perimenopause and menopause. Instead of being prepared and poised, each woman is often caught by surprise at what she experiences at every step. Sharing stories of women facing these challenges and finding healing is one way to reconnect with our collective wisdom.

A few years ago, I gathered a group of women to connect and share their stories. They ranged in age from 25 to 75. I'd been treating each of them individually with acupuncture, and what had struck me was how each one felt alone in her challenges. But I could clearly see the patterns – all the women in their 20s were facing a similar set of health and life issues, fears and uncertainties. The same was true amongst those in their 30s, 40s, 50s, 60s and 70s. In spite of the apparent increased connectivity in the age of social media, no one really felt connected to others in ways that mattered at the deeper levels. I wanted the women in each stage of life to see and hear that they were not alone, and to have women from different stages of life inform one another. The older women had wisdom and experience to share with the younger women, and the younger ones had a vibrant spirit to share with the elders.

The healing that took place in that circle of women was like a group acupuncture treatment without the needles. Indeed, it worked on the same principle: creating connection to restore balance. In this case, the connection was between individuals. Several of the younger women had suffered from depression they couldn't shake by any means. Within the first two sessions they reported that their depression had completely lifted. They felt a part of something bigger, and had received support from others who had already been through their stage of life. One of the elder women had recently lost her husband and in her grief she felt alone and unsure of what the future would hold. The younger women listened raptly to her life stories and in so doing not only were they receiving guidance, but the elder woman felt heard, relevant; she had her wisdom valued and reflected back to her in the appreciative presence and words of other women.

> *The healing that took place in that circle of women was like a group acupuncture treatment without the needles. Indeed, it worked on the same principle: creating connection to restore balance.*

In traditional cultures, women's wisdom has been passed along from one generation to the next within the community. Everyone participated in rites and rituals of passage from childhood to womanhood, through pregnancy and delivery to motherhood and through menopause. This lineage of women's wisdom is lacking in our culture today. We need to share our stories to restore it.

Acupuncture is becoming widely known for its use in supporting fertility. What isn't as well known is how acupuncture also supports each stage of pregnancy and how it can be used in labor and delivery, as well as postpartum. Because it is of interest to so many women, more in-depth information on the use acupuncture in fertility, pregnancy and postpartum has been given its own section.

## A Word About Menopause

Menopause is when the period stops. Medically, you're considered to be in menopause at the one year mark after your last period. The average age of menopause in the U.S. is 51, but it may occur earlier or later for you.

Symptoms associated with the approach of menopause may begin as many as 10 years earlier, in a phase that's called perimenopause. Some women adjust to the changes without much difficulty. But for many women, hormonal changes that start with perimenopause cause multiple symptoms that can interfere with the quality of life, including fluctuations in energy, mood, and sleep.

Perimenopausal changes can be surprising and confusing when they arise. Symptoms may include:

- Irregular menstruation
- Menorrhagia (heavy and/or prolonged periods)
- Hot flashes
- Weight gain
- Cognitive impairment/memory loss
- Loss of libido
- Anxiety
- Depression
- Palpitations
- Insomnia
- Night sweats
- Vaginal dryness
- Dry skin
- Thinning hair

Acupuncture and Chinese herbal medicine can help naturally balance you as you move through these changes, while relieving perimenopausal symptoms. Healthy diet, rest, and exercise can also be essential to your balance during these years. Some women choose to add hormone replacement therapy to help relieve unwanted symptoms. This is an individual choice to be made along with your physician. There's been a lot of misleading information about hormone replacement therapy in the media that's caused women to worry about its safety, so you have to educate yourself and be thoughtful in your decision. Read up before deciding, and try acupuncture first. Balancing your own body naturally may be preferable to moving directly into medical hormone therapy.

*The Wisdom of Menopause* by Christiane Northrup, M.D. is one of the most useful books on the subject and I recommend it for all women moving into menopause.

## Women's Healing Stories

Here are stories of women's healing using acupuncture. Within these stories, there's a full range of ailments and life situations. You will see how acupuncture treats them as parts of one whole and not as separate, unrelated symptoms.

**Renata, Age 22**
**Primary Complaint: Insomnia**
**Secondary Complaints: Anxiety, Depression, Thyroid Imbalance**
Recently graduated from college, Renata was unemployed and had severe insomnia, depression, and anxiety. Her psychiatrist had prescribed several medications including antidepressant, anti-anxiety, and sleep medications. Even with all of these, sleep was difficult and elusive. She would fall asleep around 11 p.m. with the help of medications, but woke by around 2 a.m. and remained awake until 5 or 6 a.m., when she could sometimes sleep for another hour. She was taking naps in the afternoon.

Listening to her symptoms and feeling her pulses, I sensed there was more to the story. She told me that she had suffered for a long time from an eating disorder. As a result, she was quite thin and underweight. This helped explain why such a young woman would exhibit such severe insomnia. Her body had been chronically undernourished, resulting in deficient *qi* and Blood. In Chinese medicine, the Blood is said to be "made" through the Spleen, and it is the Blood that nourishes the Heart and Liver systems to allow for healthy sleep. Extremely poor eating habits (starving herself, binging and purging) had severely weakened her digestive system. Not only had she lost vital nutrients over the course of many years, once she resumed healthy eating her digestive function was too impaired to properly handle nutrients, and she still wasn't able to build *qi* and Blood properly.

Renata had also been diagnosed with low thyroid function. Low thyroid will contribute to depression and anxiety. However, her doctor was unwilling to treat this with thyroid hormone until she had gained a sufficient amount of weight, because increased thyroid function will increase metabolism and can result in weight loss.

Within the first two treatments Renata's sleep had already improved. She was still waking up during the night, but was able to fall back to sleep with a little medication, which previously had not helped. She was overjoyed and very encouraged by this development. After a few more treatments she found that when she woke up she could fall back to sleep without any medication at all. She was gaining strength rapidly.

Renata's acupuncture treatment was aimed at restoring her digestive function so that she could begin to properly digest and metabolize her food. At the same time, I treated her to relieve the anxiety and depression and support the other systems of her body, which had been weakened over time.

Over several months of treatment, Renata gained twenty healthy pounds and developed strong muscles through her exercise program. Her doctor now agreed to give her thyroid hormone replacement, which helped support her mood and energy levels. She was sleeping through the night and enjoying more energy and a stable mood during the day. She was moving forward in her life and returning to school to become a teacher.

*Symptoms*: Insomnia, Anxiety, Depression, Low thyroid function
*Observations*: Pale tongue with red tip, weak Spleen, Blood deficiency of Heart and Liver, adrenal fatigue
*Illustrative treatment*: SP6, ST36, PC4, LI11, LV8, K3, Yintang

**Celeste, Age 32**
**Primary Complaint: Constant Pain**
**Secondary Complaints: Hopelessness, Fatigue**
At age 32, Celeste was married and had two small children. She had been in severe, constant back pain for several years. No doctor or therapy had given her any relief. Her pain radiated throughout her back but most intensely in the upper back and neck, and she had chronic headaches. When I met her, Celeste had very little hope that she could be helped, but her remaining optimism brought her to my clinic to try acupuncture.

Celeste had a very sweet, personable demeanor and a quick sense of humor, in spite of her constant pain. She told me that her husband suffered from severe, chronic depression that sometimes made him unable to work and often prevented him from getting out of bed. For her part, Celeste only felt better when she kept moving. When she sat or lay down she felt worse.

In examining Celeste I found muscle tension in her upper and lower back and neck. Internally her body was tired and showed imbalances in several systems. Her adrenal glands were depleted, not surprisingly, and there was a blockage of flow overall in both the *qi* and the Blood. This is also not surprising. It is axiomatic in Chinese medicine that "Where there is pain, there is no free flow; where there is free flow, there is no pain."

To treat Celeste effectively, we had to first get the flow of energy moving properly, by regulating the *qi* and removing stasis of Blood. We also had to help restore the adrenal system and to balance all of her systems. This would allow her body's natural healing mechanisms to kick in and start healing her from within.

At the same time, I treated the tension in the muscles of the upper and lower back and neck. In acupuncture, tired adrenals are related to weakness in the Kidneys. Deficient Kidney *qi* is associated with pain in the lower back and knees, and often radiates upward to the shoulders and neck. So the location of Celeste's pain—lower and upper back and neck—correlated with her weak Kidney *qi*. This kind of problem can be a vicious circle: stress leads to depleted Kidney *qi* and adrenal fatigue, which leads to muscle pain and tension, which further drains the Kidney *qi*. So these issues have to be treated together.

It's interesting that Celeste felt better when moving than when sitting or lying down. Since pain results from a lack of "free flow" in the body, movement is a natural remedy, and Celeste instinctively self-treated her pain with movement. Unfortunately, because of the severity of her pain syndrome, movement by itself wasn't enough to cure it, but it is a good example of the body "speaking up" about what it needs to heal. We often get clues like this through our bodies, but just as often fail to heed them. As we learn to listen to and trust our bodies' signals, we are taking a giant step toward activating our potential to self-heal.

I didn't know much about Celeste's home life, but I suspected that her husband's condition was playing a part in her pain syndrome. Because of his severe depression, she carried the weight of the family "on her shoulders," caring for the children and managing the household, while trying to cope with the effects of his depression on the family. She did not complain. All of her stress and emotional pain were expressed through the body. Did she have any other options? As far as I could see, she was doing the very best she could under very difficult circumstances. If I could help to rebalance and strengthen her body and relieve her pain, I would be doing my best to support her in whatever she needed to do to heal.

When Celeste first arrived she said she doubted anything could really help, because she had tried it all already and nothing had changed. On her second visit she commented, "I believe you can help me." This powerful statement has more to do with the essence of Chinese medicine than with me as an individual provider. Celeste had been given hope. How did it happen? This is the real "magic" of acupuncture practice: the practitioner "meets" the patient on every level—physical, mental, emotional, and spiritual. Through palpation of the body, Celeste felt that her pain has been recognized. Through a listening and aware presence, she felt that her experience was seen and felt and understood. Healing begins with presence. Sometimes presence itself is the healing. For some patients, this alone is what begins to catalyze their recovery. When combined with physical treatment, including acupuncture, massage, and other manual therapies, healing occurs at all levels of the being.

*Symptoms*: Upper and lower back pain, neck pain, headaches
*Observations*: Extreme muscle tension, deep inner fatigue and hopelessness with life situation; constrained Liver *qi*, Blood stasis, weak Spleen and Kidney *qi*, deficient Heart and Liver Blood
*Illustrative Treatment*: LV3, LI4, K7, ST36, CV6, CV12, CV17, Yintang, GB20, BL23, BL20, BL47, BL14, Trigger points: trapezius, occipitalis, supraspinatus, rhomboids, scalenes, quadratus lumborum

## Rochelle, Age 28
## Primary Complaint: Depression
## Secondary Complaints: Insomnia, Pain

Rochelle worked in advertising. She had multiple complaints and felt very "off-balance" in every way. She could not sleep and had pain all over her body. She was tired and depressed and felt very confused about what to do.

Her pulses and tongue showed Spleen deficiency, heat in the Heart, constrained Liver *qi*, impaired immune function, and deficient Blood in the Liver and Heart. All of these imbalances fit together and conspired to create her symptoms. Her pattern had developed over time, probably starting in her college days. I could guess at what those years had been like for her – working hard through school, burning the candle at both ends, then moving into the job market and working virtually night and day for the past few years. She confirmed my hunch. Her job entailed frequent travel, requiring that she catch red-eye flights to meetings and come straight back the next night and into the office without a break. All of this had weakened her adrenal glands, which are involved in the stress response, and eventually all her systems had broken down. With prolonged, relentless stress, the adrenals never get a chance to recover. It's like "running on empty," and the body cannot restore and regulate itself.

To rebalance Rochelle's body, we had to work on all of these issues simultaneously. Restoring the adrenals—part of the Kidneys in acupuncture—is fundamental. Because we're treating these glands even as the stress of life goes on, it's like putting a little fuel in the tank while the car is driving. As they get a little more energy the adrenals can begin to function better, and this supports the whole body. Ultimately, supported by the right lifestyle changes, the adrenals regain enough strength to be self-restoring.

But this isn't enough. Unless the other systems are strengthened simultaneously, the adrenals will continue to be drained and won't recover. In Rochelle's treatment, in addition to Kidney points, I used points to directly strengthen the Spleen, Liver, and Heart and to help build Blood.

> *The very first night after her initial treatment, Rochelle slept soundly for the first time in years. She felt refreshed in the morning and was noticeably happier.*

The very first night after her initial treatment, Rochelle slept soundly for the first time in years. She felt refreshed in the morning and was noticeably happier. In addition to feeling much better, she was also greatly relieved to have her condition recognized and understood. She felt she had a handle on her situation. With understanding and the right tools, she knew how to get better and no longer felt helpless and hopeless. Within a short time Rochelle was feeling strong and sleeping well consistently. Her depression had lifted and her anxiety had also gone. She continued to receive monthly treatments to help stay in balance, while modulating her schedule and adding regular exercise to her routine. She recognized that she no longer needed to work at the breakneck pace of the last ten years, and shifted gears accordingly. She saw how she could work more effectively while keeping herself in balance. This is the shift that often happens as we move from our 20s into our 30s, making life changes appropriate to longevity and balance, becoming more self-aware, and realizing that our health is central to everything else we wish to accomplish.

*Symptoms*: Insomnia, pain, depression, anxiety
*Observations*: Weak adrenals, pale tongue, constrained Liver *qi*, exhaustion, Blood deficiency
*Illustrative treatment*: K3, ST36, SP9, PC4, LV4, LV8, "Immune points," Yintang, GB20, BL23, BL20, BL14

## Charlotte: Age 43
## Primary Complaint: Itchy Skin
## Secondary Complaint: Irregular Menstruation

Charlotte was an active marketing executive, lively and vivacious. She had sought treatment because of chronic itchy skin all over her body. There was no visible rash, only the itch. She had been tested for all kinds of allergies and nothing could explain it. The doctor prescribed a medication that reduced the severity of itching by about 50 percent. But she still itched and preferred not to have to take medication every day, indefinitely.

In her detailed health history Charlotte mentioned having some problems with her period. A woman's menstrual cycle often reveals a lot about what might be underlying the primary symptoms. She said that her periods were "somewhat regular"—varying between twenty-four and thirty-two days instead of the expected twenty-eight days—and that she experienced spotting of dark blood for several days before and after. Her tongue was slightly purplish. Her pulse was thin, not as wide or full as it should be. It was also "choppy," indicating improperly regulated flow of Blood and *qi*. The irregular menstrual cycle and pattern of spotting was a sure indicator of Blood stasis. Underlying that was a deficiency of Blood.

This is not the kind of deficiency that would tend to show up on lab tests as anemia. In fact, Charlotte's blood tests were considered "normal."

Chinese medicine has tools to detect conditions that can't yet be clinically measured. Blood deficiency is often found along with Blood stasis. Even when the Blood is not truly deficient, it can appear deficient because it's not flowing properly. When the Blood is bound up in stasis and not moving well, it isn't flowing to all parts of the body where it's needed. In the skin this shortage of Blood can cause itching, as I felt it was doing in Charlotte's body. Once the Blood stasis was treated effectively and the Blood was nourished so it was no longer deficient, along with strengthening the *qi*, it was likely that her itching would also clear up.

We continued treatment for several months, with treatments every one to three weeks, with concurrent home use of medicinal herbs. Charlotte's Blood stasis was relieved and her Blood was nourished. Her period normalized to twenty-eight days without any spotting, and gradually the itching subsided and eventually cleared up completely, as expected. She no longer needed the anti-itch medication.

I didn't see Charlotte for several months. She got busy with work and travel and felt really good. When I saw her again she said she had been under a lot of stress and while doing well, was beginning to feel a hint of the itch returning. She recognized that stress was aggravating the underlying condition and that she needed to do more to stay balanced and healthy. She resolved to stop driving herself with non-stop work, leaving more time for rest and recovery. She wanted acupuncture to remain a regular part of her health program, in addition to nutrition, exercise, and rest.

It's common for people reaching their 40s to find that the lifestyle that had been working suddenly seems not to work anymore. It's bewildering at first. Our needs change as we age. We have to pay more attention to supporting our health over the long term. This does not have to be a problem—it can be an opportunity to live a healthier, much fuller life.

*Symptoms*: Unexplained itching
*Observations*: Irregular menstruation, purplish tongue, Blood deficiency and Blood stasis
*Illustrative treatment*: LV4, LV8, SP6, ST36, K6, LU7, LI11, Yintang, moxibustion, herbal supplementation

**Adrienne, Age 44**
**Primary Complaint: Hamstring Pain**
**Secondary Complaints: Anxiety, Seasonal Allergies, Weight Gain, Insomnia, Palpitations**

Adrienne was married with three children, ages 7, 11, and 14. She came in complaining of muscle tension and pain in her left hamstring, which had been bothering her for the past two-and-a-half years. Adrienne had always been an active and athletic person; she had been a competitive diver and had a good awareness of her body. She could feel a line of tension from the left side of her head down to her foot. As she described it, her left side felt tighter and her right side, weaker. She had also gained twenty pounds in the past few years that she couldn't seem to lose. Also, in the past year, her aging mother had become ill and needed a great deal of Adrienne's time and attention.

Adrienne suffered from seasonal allergies that had worsened. She had also begun to feel anxious and depressed, which she'd never felt before. The depression frightened her so much that she had taken medication to treat it.. She had decided to go off the medication by the time I saw her. Her anxiety was the biggest problem at this point, and it sometimes escalated to panic. She thought catastrophically about every ache and pain she noticed in her body and worried that it indicated a serious disease such as cancer or incipient heart attack. When her doctor heard about her palpitations along with left-sided arm pain he ordered a full set of cardiac tests. They were normal. A lot of perimenopausal women experience heart palpitations, anxiety, and chest pain and often worry they are having a heart attack when they are not. (Of course, if you think you may be having signs of a heart attack it's essential to get medical attention right away.) Because this issue is not widely discussed, it seems to each woman that she is alone in her experience.

A woman typically begins perimenopause—the hormonal changes preceding menopause—in her 40s. This coincides with the decrease in fertility that so many women over 40 are struggling with as they try to start having children at this age.

Among women in their 40s who already have children, they've typically been raising their children and taking care of the family for years while also working outside the home, which they've never had difficulty managing before. Suddenly, like Adrienne, a woman hits her mid-40s and everything seems to break down: she gains ten to twenty pounds, her aging parents need care, she develops insomnia, anxiety, depression, and fatigue, and starts getting injuries at the gym, if she manages to find the time and energy to exercise. This occurs before there are any noticeable changes to her period or hot flashes, though these may start around this time as well. When menstrual changes start, she often experiences very heavy bleeding during her periods, to the point of hemorrhage. Her heavy bleeding may go on for weeks at a time, stopping only shortly before her next period begins. This leads to anemia and fatigue and exacerbates all her other symptoms.

Adrienne's muscle tension had brought her in for acupuncture, but she was about to be treated for all the imbalances that were causing anxiety, weight gain, insomnia and allergies. In perimenopause, acupuncture rebalances the body, helping to modulate hormonal fluctuations and related symptoms. Herbal medicine often works well to provide greater support. Good nutrition and exercise are essential. Some women use natural hormonal creams such as bioidentical progesterone, applied to the skin, to help alleviate symptoms coming from hormonal fluctuations. If you're used to intense cardio workouts or running long distances, you may have to consider replacing these with some restorative yoga, walking, or other more gentle exercise, which can be a difficult adjustment to make, but essential to healing.

> *Adrienne's muscle tension had brought her in for acupuncture, but she was about to be treated for all the imbalances that were causing anxiety, weight gain, insomnia and allergies.*

Often the thyroid weakens at this time too, contributing to the fatigue, anxiety, and weight gain. Asking your medical doctor to test your thyroid may be appropriate now. Adrienne, like many women her age, felt she could not find the time to take care of all these things in addition to what she was already doing. On the other hand, she had no choice but to stop and deal with it, because she couldn't function in her current condition. She had spent her entire life putting energy out and taking care of others. It was time to take care of herself. When you lead a very full life, you have to rearrange certain priorities to restore your health—but it must be done. It is common to feel annoyed and frustrated, and possibly self-judgmental, that you're not able to keep forging ahead as you used to without having things, including your body, fall apart.

Adrienne's initial treatment left her feeling more relaxed than she had felt in years. This was visible in her face and body language. We had worked to relieve muscle tension and spasms in the neck, back, and hamstrings, and to realign both sides of her body. It was clear that she was worn out and needed deep restorative care using acupuncture while also making changes to her lifestyle.

As it happened, Adrienne was especially sensitive to the energetic movements in her body when receiving acupuncture. She was able to describe the sensation of energy moving from her left leg and hip, up her back, and over the head to the inner eye area where she had always felt "blocked." She was amazed and asked whether this could even be possible, or had she imagined it? I explained that she had just described the exact pathway of the Bladder meridian, which runs from the inner eye down the back of the body to the little toe.

Suddenly Adrienne understood that all her pains and tensions were related. Even though she didn't yet understand the "why" of it all, she had a powerful, internal awareness of her body. This helped to greatly relieve her anxiety that something more serious was wrong—that one day the doctor would confirm that she had a life-threatening illness. Sensing these interconnections helped her become even more profoundly aware of herself in relation to her body. This was the most potent healing of all for Adrienne. Informed by this awareness she could consciously choose treatments, exercises, and approaches to generate health and wellness, and assess her own progress.

Adrienne received weekly treatments for six weeks, gradually moving to twice a month and then monthly treatments as her condition improved. She incorporated appropriate gentle exercises and adjusted them as needed over time, and she began to ask for help in her life. She made positive changes to her overly busy schedule and made time to rest and restore. Her pain disappeared, her anxiety and depression cleared up, and she felt renewed energy and enthusiasm even in the midst of her many ongoing responsibilities.

*Symptoms*: Tight hamstrings, anxiety, seasonal allergies, weight gain, palpitations

*Observations*: Structural imbalance with left-sided muscle tension, constrained Liver *qi*, weak Kidney and Spleen *qi*, Heart Blood deficiency

*Illustrative treatment*: LV3, LI4, PC4, LI11, K3, K7, ST36, Yintang, BL40, BL10, BL23, BL20, BL18, BL14, Trigger points: biceps femoris, gluteus medius, quadratus lumborum, trapezius, levator scapula, supraspinatus

## Renee, Age 55
## Primary Complaint: Exhaustion
## Secondary Complaints: Stress, Back and Neck Pain

Renee was a corporate attorney, married, with two teenage sons. Five years earlier she had been diagnosed and treated for breast cancer and undergone a double mastectomy and a year of chemotherapy. She felt exhausted, with a low level of depression that she overrode with a smile and cheerful demeanor. She had come because she wanted to do something positive for herself, not knowing what she really needed.

When I examined her, I found multiple systems of weakness in Renee's body. Her adrenals were exhausted, her Spleen was weak and her Liver *qi* was constrained. Overall she presented like a "flat tire"—out of energy, out of air, just barely getting by.

I found extreme muscle tension in her neck and shoulders, which Renee hadn't even thought to mention, as she had become so accustomed to living with it. This tension can come from the strain of working at the computer all day, carrying heavy bags and, in her case, some of it was a result of the breast surgery and subsequent scar formation pulling the muscles tightly around her back. More fundamentally, the tendency for back and neck tension stemmed from her internal depletion. With no energy to hold yourself together, the muscles tighten up as if to compensate. In Chinese medicine, it's a case of internal deficiency leading to relative exterior excess (tension in the muscles). No amount of massage would relieve that tightness in the neck and back. Renee needed deep internal restoration before it would clear up.

Immediately after her first session Renee felt a lightness and happiness she hadn't felt in a long time. She slept very well that night and had more energy in the morning. It took several treatments to get more than the bare minimum of energy flowing in her system. After a month of weekly treatments, she felt like the air was back in her tires—her pulses had greater vitality and strength, and she felt more energy. It was only when she started to get energy again that Renee realized how weak and depleted she had truly been for the past five years or more. With this increased energy, her muscle tension began to relax. We built on that using gentle muscle and scar release in the neck, shoulders, back, chest and sides.

Beyond the physical healing, Renee started to get in touch with her own spirit—the part of her that kept smiling through everything, taking care of everyone but herself. She resolved to begin to speak up for herself at work and at home, and to take time for her needs as well as those of others. This was a turning point. She started by taking one hour a week for herself by coming in for treatment. She recognized that she had to become central in her own life, that she was important, that her feelings mattered, that she had her own dreams and wishes that deserved as much respect as anyone else's.

> *It was only when she started to get energy again that Renee realized how weak and depleted she had truly been for the past five years or more. With this increased energy, her muscle tension began to relax.*

*Symptoms*: Exhaustion, fatigue, flat mood, "burn-out," pain in back and neck
*Observations*: Kidney and Spleen *qi* weakness, adrenal exhaustion, constrained Liver *qi*, muscle tension in neck, shoulders, chest, sides and back, surgical scar tissue
*Illustrative treatment*: LV4, LV8, LV14, K3, ST36, PC6, LI11, CV6, CV12, CV17, Yintang, Tight, tender points: Occipitalis, cervical and upper trapezius, supraspinatus, latissimus dorsi, infraspinatus, pectoralis major

## Luciana, Age 30
## Primary Complaint: Insomnia
## Secondary Complaints: Anxiety, Shock

Luciana was married, in her first trimester of pregnancy. She worked in the fashion industry. She appeared energetic and had an engaging personality.

She had come for acupuncture to relieve her insomnia. She woke up every morning around 4 a.m. and couldn't go back to sleep. Her mind would start racing and she worried—about anything and everything. She became exhausted. In the light of day her nighttime worries seemed insignificant; at night, in bed, she found it impossible not to obsess about whatever crossed her mind—refinishing a piece of furniture or mailing a package to a family member. She recognized that her problem was not about the thing itself—it was her mind's tendency to worry and dwell that made her anxious. Anxiety was a significant problem for her throughout the day as well.

In addition to not sleeping, Luciana was experiencing the fatigue and nausea of early pregnancy.. The nausea was lifting somewhat, but she still dealt with it every day and it could be severe at times. She was weary of the pressures of her high-intensity job and wanted a change. However, she felt trapped in it.

After hearing her story, I checked Luciana's pulses and looked at her tongue. The pulses confirmed the story she had told. They showed me that Luciana had an excess of trapped energy in the Heart, combined with a weakness in her Spleen and Kidneys. There was a lack of communication between the Heart and Kidneys, a pattern that classically leads to symptoms of anxiety and insomnia. It was being exacerbated by the pregnancy, which was drawing energy from her Kidneys and Spleen. Luciana's pregnancy had intensified her symptoms and motivated her to seek help.

I often find that during pregnancy women become eager to heal and make changes in their health that are long overdue. Changes they won't or don't make for themselves, they are often eager to make for the sake of their unborn child. In this way, even the earliest stages of motherhood can begin to bring positive, transformative changes into a woman's life.

Luciana's pulses suggested to me that her body was in some kind of shock. There must have been an incident in her life that had set this pattern in motion. I asked her, "How long have you had this anxiety? What was happening in your life when it started?" She knew right away. It had started six years earlier when her brother died of cancer at a young age. Her brother's death was a huge shock to Luciana, so much so that she was unable to process her feelings about it without falling apart. So she forged ahead using a kind of brute-force determination to get through the responsibilities of her life and just to survive.

This is extremely common in cases of extreme anxiety, depression, and insomnia. A shock to the system, whether physical or emotional, often freezes us in time. It disrupts normal functioning and the beginnings of illness are set in motion. The shock and accompanying unprocessed emotions are stored in the body. Emotional memories are held in the organs, muscles, connective tissue, and other cells. These unprocessed emotions may lead to serious illness over time.

> *A shock to the system, whether physical or emotional, often freezes us in time. It disrupts normal functioning and the beginnings of illness are set in motion.*

Initially this is often a survival mechanism: when an event is too much to process in the moment, the body will "store" it for us. The problem is that we never get back to it. Unprocessed emotion stored in the body is its own kind of "germ." Because we are not able to let it out (we don't know how, and eventually we forget it was ever there), the body and mind cannot function properly. The energy flow is blocked. It's like what happens when a dam forms in the midst of a flowing river: the river's flow is blocked, and water has to find ways around it. But as hard as it tries, there will still be blocked water that pools above the dam and may even become stagnant. A new ecosystem is formed and changes the entire environment. This is what happens in the body when our internal flow is blocked in some way.

In the simplest terms, healing through acupuncture is about removing blockages to allow the body to heal itself. In one sense, all illness

> *In the simplest terms, healing through acupuncture is about removing blockages to allow the body to heal itself.*

traces back to the blockage or impairment of normal functioning. When we remove that blockage and provide the right support, the body has the power to heal itself.

In treating Luciana that first day, I used acupuncture points to relieve blocked energy and begin to re-establish proper communication between her different body systems. I could tell from the change in her pulse qualities that it had worked. Luciana left the treatment hopeful for change, knowing that she could not go on in the way she had been living.

When I saw her the next week, Luciana was effusive in communicating her delight over the effects of her initial treatment. Not only had she slept through the night for six nights straight—the previous night was the only time she had woken up at 4 a.m.—but her nausea was now only very mild and infrequent.

When your body has held a pattern of imbalance for a long time, it needs a series of acupuncture treatments to coax and support it to regain and sustain the new state of balance. During the initial treatment, rebalancing begins. The effects of that treatment will tend to be strongest over the next 24-72 hours, and up to a week, depending on the severity of the condition. How long the benefits last is one indicator that we use to determine how frequently to provide subsequent treatments. It's expected that treatments will occur more frequently at first and less often over time as the body becomes better able to hold its new state of balance. In Luciana's case, her sleep was good for six days and only the day before her next scheduled acupuncture treatment she'd had a bout of insomnia again. This is typical in the healing process. It was time for another acupuncture treatment.

Luciana's pulses suggested that there had been some very positive changes in her body and yet we still had work to do.

During treatment, after placing the acupuncture needles in the selected points, it's common to give the body time to assimilate the changes we are setting in motion. Some people are uncomfortable with the idea of just lying on the treatment table alone during this time. Luciana expressed this anxiety, saying she didn't know how to be alone with her own mind. She was usually engaged in some activity: working, checking email, talking on the phone—anything to avoid being quiet by herself. A lot of people sense this inner disquiet and know something's wrong but they're not quite sure what it is. They say, as Luciana did, "I could never meditate. My mind is uncontrollable."

The mind is in the habit of spinning out of control with thoughts when you're left alone, trying to fend off the stored emotions, which would be overwhelming to feel — or so you believe. It's as if you've hidden a monster in your closet and as long as there's activity in the house you won't hear its cries to get out. But if the house becomes quiet you're going to hear it screaming. Our stored emotions are like that monster. We drown out its cries with some other kind of noise.

As a result we become scared of our own mind, of being alone, or of just being quiet. The tragedy is that it's in our quietude that we access our greatest resources for healing, wellness, and living life fully. We've not only locked up the monster in the closet but also our truest selves. To heal, and to live life fully and authentically, the part of ourselves that we've locked away needs to be released.

Acupuncture tends to gently induce a meditative state in the body and mind, and this is part of its power to heal. The nervous system becomes balanced and the whole body is harmonized. The blood pressure and body temperature naturally drop, and a state of relaxation is induced. Many people enter a peaceful state of rest or fall asleep. This can give you a head start if you want to learn to meditate. Once you've felt this experience in your own body it's easier to know what you're aiming for, and to understand the benefits that the practice of meditation can provide.

> *Acupuncture tends to gently induce a meditative state in the body and mind, and this is part of its power to heal. The nervous system becomes balanced and the whole body is harmonized.*

Luciana arrived at her next visit with tremendous clarity about her life's direction. She had decided that she would remain at her current job until the baby was born, and after taking time for maternity leave, she would seek a new job, more to her liking. She and her husband had also decided to look for a new home, in preparation for the baby—something she had been afraid to do before. She was no longer fearful of making these changes, and knowing she had a plan was already making it so much easier to go to work every day.

This clarity and ability to plan was a clear sign that Luciana was healing. The same blocked physical energy that had created anxiety and insomnia was keeping her mind and spirit from moving as well. As the blocked energy started to move, she felt the benefits at every level of her life, which opened many new doors. She found solutions she had never before considered. Luciana came in for insomnia and within a few weeks had found an entirely new perspective of hope and optimism for her life.

*Symptoms*: Insomnia, anxiety, nausea and fatigue in early pregnancy
*Observations*: Emotional shock, constrained Liver *qi*, weakened Spleen and Kidney *qi*, trapped *qi* and heat in the Heart
*Illustrative treatment*: LV3, PC6, LI11, K4, K27, SP9, Yintang

**Arielle: Age 28**
**Primary Complaint: Foot Pain**
**Secondary Complaint: Unresolved Grief**

Arielle worked in banking and was very accomplished for her age. She exuded a quality of warmth, happiness, and maturity. Her aunt had told her that acupuncture had alleviated her own back pain when nothing else had helped, so Arielle thought she'd try it for the toes of her right foot, which had gone numb. She was a runner who had trained and run in a marathon the previous year, but by the time the foot pain started she was running less, so it seemed strange to her that it started when it did. She hoped the injury and numbness in her foot wouldn't involve any permanent nerve damage.

As I examined Arielle I found structural imbalance that was probably putting too much pressure on the toes when she walked. Arielle confirmed that she had pain in her left lower back and hip. With her hip pulled up due to muscle tension on the left side, her right foot was striking the ground in a way that put undue pressure on her right toes. That pressure was squeezing nerves supplying the toes, causing them go numb. I didn't think the damage was permanent, although nerves can be slower to recover than other systems in the body. I gave her treatment to restore balance in the back, hips, pelvis, and legs to take the pressure off the toe. I recommended that she support the treatment with appropriate stretches and exercises to retain a healthy structural balance. I anticipated that the numbness in her toes would improve over several months' time, once the structural imbalance was corrected.

Internally Arielle's body was weak and tired. She didn't have enough energy and also suffered from Blood deficiency, which itself can contribute to numbness. So while her structure was putting too much pressure on her toes, her Blood deficiency was making her more prone to experience numbness as a result. Restoring healthy sensation to the toes would include treating the Blood deficiency as well.

Arielle's Blood deficiency was related to a weakness in the Spleen, which includes aspects of digestion, lymphatic fluid, and immunity. If the Spleen is weak, you won't be able to optimize the nutrition you take in, even if you're eating a healthy diet. The Spleen is easily weakened due to overthinking, worry, eating too fast and on the go (over meetings or the computer for example), eating too much cold and raw food, drinking too many cold drinks, and letting too much time pass between meals. Most of us are guilty of this to one degree or another. Spleen weakness is very common. And one absolute sign of it is fatigue.

Arielle also had signs in her pulse indicating that some kind of shock had occurred in her life. I asked her about it and without hesitation she knew exactly when it had happened. Six years ago her twin sister had died in a car accident. Her mother suffered from severe depression for which she had been repeatedly hospitalized, and her father had left when the children were young, with no word of his whereabouts. All of these life circumstances, along with the trauma of her sister's tragic death, had put Arielle into a state of shock.

Arielle's mother had never really been present for her, due to her own illness, so she had missed out on the essential nurturing that a mother provides from the earliest days of life and throughout childhood. Without such mothering and nurturance, the Spleen wasn't able to really develop properly, and she most likely started out with a weakness in that system which was compounded over time. Arielle agreed that she often felt fatigued, but she thought it was just to be expected with her busy lifestyle and long work hours.

As soon as I acknowledged Arielle's trauma and pain by telling her what I was seeing in her body, she began to cry. That may seem unremarkable except that she told me—over and over—how strange it was. "I never cry," she said. The lack of crying after all that she had endured was one of the signs of shock in her body, mind and spirit. The shock froze her emotions, which were too strong to process at the time, especially given her lack of mothering throughout childhood. By freezing up, Arielle could feel more certain of her ability to cope and survive. It is a reasonable short-term solution that turns into a long-term dysfunction, and ultimately, illness.

Arielle was amazed that though she had consulted me for the numbness in her toes, so much more had been revealed and opened up and begun to heal. She said she had been afraid to feel her pain because she thought she might be unable to cope with daily living. We talked about letting it out in a controlled and guided way, like letting the steam out of a pressure cooker a little at a time, not opening the lid all at once. She felt very encouraged by this possibility. As we continued acupuncture treatments over the next couple of months, Arielle's energy increased, her back and hip pain disappeared, and the numbness in her toes completely disappeared.

*Symptoms*: Numb toes, fatigue
*Observations*: Structural imbalance in lower back, pelvis, and legs, weak Spleen, Blood deficiency, emotional shock
*Illustrative treatment*: SP3, ST36, LI11, PC 6, LV 8, K3, local points between toes on top of foot, Yintang, BL20, BL13, Trigger points: gluteus medius, piriformis, lumbar paraspinals, quadratus lumborum

## Sophie, Age 32
## Primary Complaint: Depression
## Secondary Complaints: Fatigue, Shock

Sophie was a successful attorney who nonetheless suffered from chronic, long-term depression and low energy. She struggled to get up in the morning and carry out her daily responsibilities. At the end of the day she would go home and collapse in front of the television and then go to sleep. Her pulses revealed several patterns of imbalance that would explain the fatigue and depression. I asked her when the depression had started. She said it began at age 14 and had been relentless ever since. "Was there anything you remember happening at that age that was upsetting or unsettling?" I asked. "Did you move or change schools?" Sophie said her parents had divorced when she was 14 and this had been an emotional shock. She felt vulnerable and afraid and didn't have the emotional tools to cope with her feelings. Her parents were wrapped up in their own divorce and were unavailable to help her deal with her own loss.

I often see conditions of depression and anxiety that seem to be rooted in a childhood emotional trauma of some kind. Trauma in childhood can easily occur in response to events that no adult would even identify as problematic. It can come from a family move, bullying, a sibling's injury or accident, a bike accident, as well as from more obvious stressors like parental divorce or death. A trauma at any age that isn't resolved can lead to patterns of illness in the body, mind, and emotions. When it happens in childhood it can be harder to treat as an adult, because the trauma was frozen and trapped within a child's sensibilities, making it more difficult to access and resolve.

In a case like Sophie's, psychotherapy can be helpful, but its usefulness will tend to be limited until the shock is cleared from the body. An adult patient may develop a rational understanding of her problem, yet still feel stuck in it. Similarly, if I treated Sophie for her depression and fatigue using acupuncture, without first clearing the shock, the results would be limited. She might feel a bit better but would require ongoing treatment to maintain only a slight improvement in her condition. So the first step was to clear the shock in the body, which we did. After that, using acupuncture and psychotherapy in conjunction brought Sophie significant lasting relief from depression and fatigue.

*Symptoms*: Depression, fatigue and lethargy
*Observations*: Emotional shock from childhood, weak Spleen and Kidney *qi*, Liver *qi* constraint
*Illustrative treatment*: LV3, PC6, LI11, CV6, CV12, CV17, SP6, ST36, Yintang

## Norah, Age 50
## Primary Complaint: Lower Back and Knee Pain
## Secondary Complaints: Chronic Sinusitis, Weight Gain, Perimenopause

Norah was a single mother of a 9-year-old boy when she first came for acupuncture. She complained of lower back and knee pain. She worked, seated, for long hours at her desk, which worsened the condition. Her secondary complaint was chronic sinusitis. Third, she complained of being about 25 pounds overweight. Before having her child at age 41, she was 25 pounds lighter, exercised regularly and felt healthy and fit. Like so many parents of young children, becoming a mother meant her own health routine went out the window. She no longer exercised, made poor food choices, and was constantly tired.

In the acupuncture diagnosis I felt Norah's pulses, looked at her tongue, and felt pressure points on her abdomen and on the arms, legs, knees, and back. Although she had consulted me about back and knee pain, I needed to know more about her overall balance and state of health before treating her. Chronic sinus conditions are almost always associated with a weakness in the Spleen, which I found in Norah. Her body type (fleshy and pale), fatigue, tongue's appearance, and pulse qualities all showed a Spleen deficiency. In such cases the body tends to produce phlegm, which then appears in the upper respiratory system, including the sinus cavities. There was swelling of the sinus tissue and inflammation that, along with the phlegm, had led to a chronic state of sinusitis. A person with this pattern is often clearing the throat because of post-nasal sinus drip, which worsens just after eating. They may also wake up in the morning with a dull headache from the building of pressure in the sinuses overnight.

At age 50 Norah was also in the later stages of perimenopause. Her periods were irregular and she suffered from occasional hot flashes. Women's hormones go through many changes as they pass through perimenopause into menopause, and adrenal fatigue is often an important factor. If you've been living a stressful life for many years, at perimenopause and menopause the adrenal system, already stressed, is going to be strained even further. The same chemical building blocks that make up adrenal hormones also make up our reproductive hormones. Therefore, when the reproductive hormone levels begin to fluctuate in perimenopause, there is often a concomitant strain on the adrenals. Multiple symptoms begin to arise "out of nowhere" as the body seems to start falling apart.

Healthy adrenals play a role in our stress response. Their influence helps maintain balance in many other systems throughout the body. They provide the body with its own natural anti-inflammatory ability and help regulate metabolism and body weight, among other things. Norah's inflammation – which her weakened adrenals had difficulty fighting

– played a part in her sinus condition as well as in the arthritis in her lumbar spine and knees.

In acupuncture, the adrenals are part of the Kidneys, which include aspects of the endocrine system as well as the kidneys and bladder. The Kidneys are the storehouse of our underlying reserve energy supply. Just as we may have a full or overdrawn bank account, our Kidney energy may be abundant or very weak. We drain this "reserve account" by living beyond our energetic means for long

*Norah's inflammation – which her weakened adrenals had difficulty fighting – played a part in her sinus condition as well as in the arthritis in her lumbar spine and knees.*

periods of time. It also naturally tends to become weaker as we age. Most of the signs of aging can be attributed to the Kidneys. One classic sign of weak Kidneys is low back and knee pain.

The key to treating Norah's back and knee pain is best understood in light of her whole story. She gave birth in her 40s, at a stage in life when the Kidneys are already in decline. Subsequently she exhausted herself taking care of her baby, losing sleep, dropping her exercise routine and beginning to consume more sugar, junk food, and caffeine to give her a feeling of energy, all the while continuing to work full-time. She was by now drinking a lot of wine to relieve her stress, "probably more than is good for me," she said.

Treating Norah's back and knee pain was relatively straightforward using acupuncture. The knees were aching but had no significant damage, and the pain in her back was coming from compressed and inflamed discs. Acupuncture treats this kind of pain and inflammation very well.

To really treat her back and knee pain successfully, we had to treat the underlying imbalances, primarily those in the Kidneys and Spleen. This is known as treating both the "root and branch" of illness. The root of Norah's condition was the underlying depletion, and the branches were the symptoms: the pain and inflammation in the back, knees, and sinuses. Within a few treatments Norah's back and knee pain were virtually gone, her energy level was much higher, and her sinuses had improved significantly. She had naturally reduced her wine intake as her energy and mood improved and made an effort to eat healthier, wholesome foods that could be prepared simply and quickly.

*Symptoms*: Lower back and knee pain, weight gain, sinusitis, hot flashes, fatigue
*Observations*: Fleshy body, pale skin, weak Spleen and Kidneys, adrenal fatigue, inflammation
*Illustrative treatment*: K3, K7, SP9, ST36, LV4, LU5, LI11, Local sinus points on the face, BL23, BL20, BL18, BL13, GB20, Tight, tender points on lower and upper back and around the sacrum, moxibustion

## Catherine, Age 53
### Primary Complaint: Sinusitis and Chronic Sinus Infection
### Secondary Complaint: Fatigue

Catherine was an energetic mother of five who worked as a high-level executive. She traveled frequently for work. She'd always had high energy but for the past four months had suffered from a severe sinus infection that was unresponsive to multiple rounds of antibiotic treatment.

Catherine's sinus congestion was extreme. She couldn't breathe through her nose and when speaking she sounded like she had a severe cold. Her pulses and other body signs indicated Spleen weakness, with excess phlegm in the Lungs, adrenal fatigue, deficiency heat, and Liver *qi* constraint.

Acupuncture treatment focused on restoring strength to the depleted Spleen and adrenals, helping her body's energy flow freely, and clearing the phlegm. In addition to body points on the arms and legs, some local acupuncture points were used around the sinus areas in the head to clear the inflammation and congestion there.

Usually, a case this severe would require a series of treatments to fully clear the sinusitis. Sinus conditions can be stubborn at first and require lifestyle support through dietary choices, nasal rinses (saline spray or neti pot irrigation), and sometimes herbs, used internally or topically. In Catherine's case, the response was surprisingly immediate and dramatic. By the next day, her sinus congestion was relieved considerably, and over the next week it cleared up completely.

*Symptoms*: Sinus congestion and infection, fatigue
*Observations*: weak Spleen *qi*, adrenal fatigue, inflammation, heat in the Lungs and phlegm
*Illustrative treatment*: SP3, ST40, ST36, LI11, "Immune points," LU7, LI4, K7, GB20, Yintang, local facial points for the sinus

### Ginny, Age 55
### Primary Complaint: Asthma
### Secondary Complaint: Immune System Weakness

Every year in the summer Ginny suffered from extreme attacks of asthma, requiring life-saving medication and occasional hospitalization.

Ginny told me that these bouts of asthma had been occurring for several years. Her family vacation home was a cottage in the mountains where they went every summer, and visits there always made her asthma worse. She believed the mold in the cottage had triggered her asthma.

Feeling her pulses and examining the signs on her body, I could tell that Ginny's adrenals were stressed and fatigued and her immune system was also strained. We started treatment in July—in the midst of her most symptomatic season. Her Spleen, Kidneys, and Lungs were very weak, combining to create deficient heat that expressed as inflammation and together created her asthma symptoms.

With acupuncture treatment, Ginny felt immediate relief from her wheezing and shortness of breath. Even so, there was a long way to go before her body was fully balanced, strengthened, and restored. I encouraged her to continue treatment beyond the point of immediate symptom relief. She followed my advice up to a point, coming weekly for treatment for about six weeks. I felt there was still more work needed to balance her body, but she felt completely better and so she stopped coming for treatment. Because her symptoms became severe every year in June and July, I recommended that Ginny return for acupuncture in the winter or early spring to boost her system in advance of the summer. However, I didn't see her again until the following July, when her asthma once again flared up. She returned for several weekly treatments until her asthma was again under control.

In Ginny's case, the best acupuncture approach would be to treat her far beyond the point where she feels the relief of asthma symptoms. This is difficult for many people to do, because they feel better and life's other demands take priority over making time for acupuncture treatment. While acupuncture does a great job of symptom relief, its even greater strength is in its ability to fortify and balance the body so that it can fight off illness on its own.

*Symptoms*: Wheezing, shortness of breath, fatigue
*Observations*: red tongue, rapid, weak pulse, adrenal exhaustion, inflammation, immune stress
*Illustrative treatment*: K6, K27, LU7, "Immune points," LI11, ST36, SP9, LI4

## Leigh, Age 45
### Primary Complaint: Tinnitus
### Secondary Complaints: Migraines, Allergies

Leigh came to acupuncture for ringing in her ears. She sometimes suffered from migraines. She had been to the doctor, who suggested that she try acupuncture. She was very worried, as she had heard that tinnitus – ringing in the ears – was hard to cure, and she could not imagine having to live with it forever.

Ear ringing is a common affliction and it can range from mild to extreme. In acupuncture, there are different types of ear ringing coming from either deficiency or excess. In a separate category is injury—hearing that has been impaired through infection or loud noises. The type of ringing it is determines the way it is treated with acupuncture, as well as the prognosis.

> *She was very worried, as she had heard that tinnitus – ringing in the ears – was hard to cure, and she could not imagine having to live with it forever.*

Leigh's pulses and tongue revealed a pattern of Spleen deficiency with phlegm, and weakness of the immune system. There was constraint in the Liver and some degree of weakness in the Kidneys as well, probably due to prolonged stress. In Leigh's case, part of that stress was commuting two to three hours daily to and from work. She was also suffering from allergies—the ultimate cause of her ear ringing—and this too was an ongoing internal stress. We often conceive of stress as unpleasant emotional tension, but stress can come from internal sources as well, including allergy and infection. It can come from extra-long days of work or exertion of any kind, including fun activities. Stress takes many forms and isn't always experienced as unpleasant.

I treated Leigh weekly for several months. During this time her migraines cleared up and her ear ringing resolved completely. At first, the symptoms would recede and then return. Leigh began to notice that her ringing came back on the weekends and started to realize that there was something at home causing an allergic reaction, to which her body would respond with ear ringing and a migraine. It would worsen over the weekends when she was home for two days. The body's allergic reaction created congestion in her head and ears that impeded circulation and prevented lymphatic drainage. This in turn created imbalance and an actual physical pressure that led to headache and ear ringing symptoms. She proceeded to remove old carpets and replace her bedding to reduce the chance of allergens in her home environment. As her internal systems were balanced through acupuncture and she cleared the home of allergens, Leigh's ear ringing healed completely.

Ear ringing that comes with age and injury is less responsive to treatment with acupuncture. If there has been nerve damage due to infection or loud noises, it is generally very difficult to resolve. Age-related impaired hearing and tinnitus can often be incrementally but not substantially improved using acupuncture.

*Symptoms*: Ears ringing, migraines, sinus congestion
*Observations*: weak Spleen and Kidney *qi*, Liver *qi* constraint, immune system weakness, phlegm obstruction
*Illustrative treatment*: SP3, ST40, GB20, TH17, LV3, LI4, LU7, "Immune points," K7, K27, Yintang, Bi tang

## Carla, Age 45
## Primary Complaint: Vertigo
## Secondary Complaint: Stress

Carla, a journalist and mother of three, felt healthy and energetic in spite of her demanding schedule. But she suffered from vertigo. It would come and go, and was worse with sudden movements of the head or when lying down and sitting up. She had been to an ear, nose, and throat doctor who had diagnosed a "benign condition of unknown origin." There was no medical treatment suggested.

When I felt Carla's pulses and assessed the body's signs, I found excess phlegm, probably generated by a deficient Spleen, and constraint in the Liver leading to a lack of regulation and smooth flow in the body. There seemed to be a structural component as well, and in taking her history I learned that Carla had suffered a rather severe head injury, falling and hitting the back of her head. My assessment was that the head injury caused a structural imbalance leading to blockage in the region of the neck and head. This meant that there could be physical compression of the bones, muscles, and fascia in the area, causing restricted flow of blood and lymph. This in turn could lead to impaired function in that region and probable compression of the nerves that regulate balance.

Acupuncture treatment involved restoring harmony in the internal systems of the Spleen and Liver, eliminating phlegm, and relieving the physical compression and restricted flow in the head and ear area.

To do this, acupuncture needles were placed in points on the arms and legs, and also in the area of the neck and head around the ears to directly relieve the structural constraint and tension. Carla received weekly acupuncture treatments for four weeks, after which her vertigo was completely relieved.

*Symptoms*: Vertigo
*Observations*: weak Spleen with phlegm, Liver *qi* constraint, structural imbalance, history of head injury
*Illustrative treatment*: LV3, LI4, TH9, K9, SP9, ST36, GB20, GB8, ST8

## Erika, Age 35
## Primary Complaint: Interstitial Cystitis
## Secondary Complaint: Anxiety

At the time of her first visit Erika was the mother of two young children. The baby was 8 months old. She had come for treatment in desperation due to severe urinary symptoms and pain, which had been going on for about seven weeks. At her recent doctor's visit she was examined and told that there was no detectable urinary tract infection.

Just in case there might be some infection that was undetectable, she was given a month's supply of antibiotics, along with some pain medication. Neither medication had any effect. Her doctors suggested that she might have interstitial cystitis (IC). When she read about it online, Erika found it described as a chronic inflammation of the bladder wall that can't be explained due to other causes, such as infection or urinary stones. There is no definitive test for IC and medical treatment tends to be focused on coping and pain management. There is no known cure.

Erika was in constant burning pain that was so severe it woke her up at night. Urination was frequent and painful. She was also exhausted from lack of sleep, which is an issue for all mothers of babies but was made worse by her inability to sleep due to pain.

Over the years, she had suffered from repeated bouts of UTIs and took a prophylactic antibiotic before sex to help reduce the chances of infection. This recent bout was the worst she had experienced, and it began within months of giving birth to her second child. In addition to being in severe pain, Erika was emotionally distraught. A diagnosis of IC can mean a lifetime of pain management for many people.

Examination of Erika's pulse, tongue, and pressure points revealed the internal pattern of disharmony behind her painful condition, one of fire in the Liver, Kidney, and Heart along with a deficiency in the Spleen and a weakened immune system. She also had severe muscle tension in the lower abdomen and deep pelvic muscles, which had to be cleared up using trigger-point release.

Using the appropriate points along the affected meridians and releasing the chronic muscle spasms, along with some herbal therapy, Erika felt immediate relief leading to complete resolution of the problem within a couple of months. She has remained pain-free since then, even through a third pregnancy and childbirth.

*Symptoms*: Severe bladder pain, burning, frequent, urgent urination
*Observations*: Inflammation, Spleen and Immune system weakness, fire in Liver, Kidney and Heart meridians, repeated urinary tract infections and antibiotic use, two pregnancies and deliveries, chronic muscle spasms in lower abdomen and pelvis

*Illustrative treatment*: K7, K10, LV4, LV8, ST36, LI11, PC4, CV3, CV12, CV17, ST 28, Yintang, BL23, BL28, BL43, Trigger points: piriformis, deep pelvic muscles, lower abdominal muscles, herbal therapy at home

## Kimberly, Age 34
## Primary Complaint: Chronic, Recurrent Urinary Tract Infection
## Secondary Complaint: Sexual Dysfunction and Pain

Kimberly arrived for acupuncture complaining of chronic urinary tract infection that had been unresponsive to antibiotics. Her medical tests confirmed that she did have an infection, but it was resistant to treatment with every known antibiotic. She'd had several rounds of kidney infections with severe lower back pain and copious blood in her urine. She followed every good hygiene practice she knew, including showering after sex, and she didn't have any anatomical anomaly, such as a shortened urethra. Her symptoms varied somewhat with her menstrual cycle, so for two weeks out of each month it felt a bit better. It was difficult for her to have sex with her husband due to the pain and as a result their sexual intimacy had suffered, causing stress for both of them. She said that her husband was very understanding and supportive.

She told me she had suffered from this chronic UTI for four years. "What else happened four years ago?" I asked. "Four years ago I gave birth to my son," she said. Hearing this, I felt confident that we would be able to clear up Kimberly's chronic UTI completely. Even before checking her pulse, her history told me that most likely childbirth had left her pelvic region with chronic muscle spasms that led to inadequate nerve and blood supply to the region. The area was in distress. Yes, she did have an infection in the urinary tract which was not responding to antibiotics. For the purposes of healing, we first needed to restore full function to the lower abdomen, pelvis, and urinary tract while strengthening her immune system. By making the area strong, the urinary tract would no longer be susceptible to harboring infection.

I used acupuncture points on the arms and legs to help restore balance to Kimberly's internal systems, along with trigger point release on the lower abdomen, lower back, and deep pelvic muscles of the buttocks to relieve the chronic muscle tension in these areas and restore healthy flow of blood, lymph, and nerve function.

Urinary tract problems are often diagnosed in Chinese medicine as heat or fire in the lower burner. Sometimes there is also a condition of dampness, which can be found with stones or with genital infections like vaginal yeast or herpes. In each case, an essential part of the treatment involves resolving the condition of heat, fire, or dampness. In doing this, we're changing the underlying environment that allows an infection to thrive there. This is a key element in Chinese medicine: not only do you treat the symptom or offending infection, as with antibiotics and many other Western medications—you change the environment itself.

Within a few treatments Kimberly's symptoms had cleared up almost completely and she had discontinued antibiotic use, while supplementing with probiotics instead. She came for weekly acupuncture treatments for another month, at which point she had no remaining pain with sex or at any stage of her menstrual cycle—and no infection.

*Symptoms*: Chronic, recurrent urinary tract infections, sexual dysfunction and pain

*Observations*: Urinary tract problems started after childbirth, subsequent kidney infections with blood in the urine, chronic muscle spasms in lower abdomen and pelvis

*Illustrative treatment*: K7, K10, LV 4, LV8, SP9, ST36, LI11, "Immune points," PC4, CV3, ST28, Trigger points: lower abdominal and pelvic muscles

## Toni, Age 52
## Primary Complaint: Shoulder Pain
## Secondary Complaints: Constipation, Herpes, Thyroid Imbalance, Perimenopause

Toni was a 52-year-old artist who came in for treatment of shoulder pain. She also suffered from fatigue and constipation. She'd just had an outbreak of genital herpes, for the first time in over twenty years. "Why now?," she asked. Nothing had significantly changed lately—she had been married to her husband for 20 years, her job was unchanged, there was no new stress in her life. However, like everyone, Toni did have stress, and she managed it, she told me, by drinking "too much" wine, up to a full bottle every night.

Upon examination, I found that Toni's pattern was one of dampness and heat, along with deficiency in the Kidneys and Spleen. Her doctor was treating her for a hypothyroid condition, and she was taking thyroid hormone medication. She was still menstruating, but not regularly, as she was in the later stage of perimenopause.

Toni's condition also involved adrenal depletion, exacerbated by the hormonal changes of late perimenopause, along with a weakness in the digestive and immune systems. The Kidneys in Chinese medicine encompass aspects of the endocrine or hormonal system. When this system weakens with age, combined with perimenopause, women frequently begin to have outright symptoms of thyroid insufficiency and start taking thyroid hormone replacement, as Toni was doing. Particularly when there is thyroid insufficiency in perimenopause, there is often also adrenal fatigue. This is a depletion of the Kidneys and can often lead to a combination of both heat and cold symptoms in the body. The hypothyroid condition is a kind of cold condition (some of its key signs are a tendency to feel cold and have cold hands and feet). The adrenal fatigue, on the other hand, leads to a kind of heat, which is primarily considered a "deficiency heat" condition, meaning the heat arises out of deficiency. Hot flashes may occur as a symptom associated with this mix of imbalances. Because of her weak Spleen and high alcohol consumption, Toni had also developed internal damp heat, particularly in the Liver. All of these factors together create the perfect conditions for an outbreak of genital herpes.

Medical science knows that the herpes simplex virus "hides" in the nerves once a person has been infected and emerges under various stressful conditions. Some people use antiviral medications to curb an outbreak and prophylactically to avoid future outbreaks. Others take lysine, an amino acid that can help prevent outbreaks if taken regularly, while avoiding arginine-rich foods. Beyond that, reducing stress and supporting the immune system is the best preventive measure you can take.

Acupuncture goes one step further. By looking at the internal imbalances in the body we can restore a healthy environment that is less conducive to a viral outbreak. That is just what we did in Toni's case. Using acupuncture, we balanced the meridians that were out of balance due to her stage of life and the hormonal changes. We used acupuncture and herbs to clear the internal dampness and heat and to balance the affected meridians. I strongly advised her to curtail her alcohol use, which was contributing to the condition.

As Toni's original complaints had included shoulder pain and constipation, we worked with these conditions at the same time. When we address underlying imbalances, very often multiple seemingly unrelated symptoms resolve simultaneously. Toni's internal heat, combined with the underlying Spleen and Kidney *qi* deficiency, were contributing to the symptom of constipation. Interestingly, Toni's shoulder pain was located in muscles along the Small and Large Intestine meridians. Along with treating the internal imbalances, I released trigger points located in the muscles of the shoulder. We created a nutritional program to support her intestines and digestion. Using diet, acupuncture, lifestyle changes and herbs, we were able to resolve Toni's hot flashes, her energy level increased, her stress decreased (as well as her alcohol consumption), her constipation cleared up, and the shoulder pain was gone as well. This whole process took about eight weeks of weekly treatments.

*Symptoms*: Shoulder pain, constipation, herpes, fatigue, hot flashes
*Observations*: dampness, heat, weak Spleen and Kidney *qi*, hormonal imbalance, immune system weakness, Liver *qi* constraint, excessive alcohol consumption
*Illustrative treatment*: LI15, TH4, K6, LU7, SP9, LV5, ST36, SI10, Yintang, Trigger points of shoulder region: deltoid, teres minor, coracobrachialis, triceps

## Natalie, Age 30
### Primary Complaint: Painful Periods (Dysmenorrhea)
### Secondary Complaints: Headache, Back Pain, Unresolved Grief

Natalie, a graphic designer, came for acupuncture because of headaches and back pain that accompanied painful menstrual periods. She also said she felt "out of whack" and wanted to get balanced overall. In addition, she was tired of her job and no longer felt challenged by it, but wasn't sure what to do. Five years earlier her mother had died, at a time when Natalie was just getting started in her career and independent life as a young adult. She didn't know what to do except to keep pushing through. She never really had the time or a way of grieving and processing her loss.

Grieving is a process of releasing and letting go. It's inherent in life because everything is transient and constantly changing. Nothing is static. You can never reach the perfect state of balance and simply lock it in. Because life is in a perpetually dynamic state of flux, achieving wellness involves ongoing, conscious rebalancing. It involves all of our "parts"—not just the physical body, but also our mind, emotions, and spirit.

Grief is associated with the Lungs and Large Intestine. These two organs comprise the metal element. With our Lungs we inhale oxygen-rich air and exhale deoxygenated air in a continuous cycle of receiving and letting go. Similarly, the Large Intestine is the final step in digestion where we hold onto vital water and nutrients, and release the body's waste. Here again, we're taking in and holding that which supports life, and releasing the part we no longer need. Grief is the emotional expression of this process of letting go of what we no longer have or need.

Even though we notice it most with our greatest losses, grief is a part of daily life in many smaller ways each time we have to let go of anything – an idea, a desired outcome, that cup of coffee you wanted but couldn't have. To learn to grieve well is to learn to live in balance with the dynamic state of flux that is life. Unresolved grief remains frozen within us and can block our growth and make us ill. Because every system in our body is interdependent, if one part becomes frozen and stuck, others will eventually suffer as well.

> *To learn to grieve well is to learn to live in balance with the dynamic state of flux that is life. Unresolved grief remains frozen within us and can block our growth and make us ill. Because every system in our body is interdependent, if one part becomes frozen and stuck, others will eventually suffer as well.*

Natalie was feeling "out of whack," fatigued, with a lot of back pain and headaches, which pointed to some blockage she couldn't define. Instinctively she knew that all her symptoms were connected to something more fundamental, but she didn't know what that was. She hoped that acupuncture would help.

In her first acupuncture treatment Natalie relaxed and then, unexpectedly, she started to sob on the table. She thought of her mother and how much she missed her. She began to make conscious the grief that had been frozen inside and left incompletely resolved. Not only did her physical pain vanish, but she began to feel the freedom to take the next steps in her life, to seek a new job, to let her creative skills flourish, to dream and plan her life the way she truly wanted to live it.

Natalie continued treatment over several months to fully relieve her muscle tension and other patterns of blockage: trigger points in the back, neck, and shoulders, as well as in the abdomen; headaches; Blood stasis and dysfunction of energy flow causing premenstrual symptoms and painful periods. Each month her PMS lessened until it disappeared completely, and her periods became virtually pain-free.

While PMS and painful periods have come to be seen as "normal" by most women, it is more accurate to say they are "common." With acupuncture it is entirely possible to be free from premenstrual and menstrual discomfort. Any stress, fatigue, injury or illness that causes even a slight impairment of blood flow through the uterus becomes a blockage that leads to even greater blockage of flow, like water stuck behind a dam. Even a small blockage can grow quickly due to the volume of blood the body is trying to move. Where there is blockage, there is pain; when that blockage is removed, pain is relieved as well. For women with menstrual pain or irregularities, receiving acupuncture once or twice a month is an effective way to keep the menstrual cycle healthy, and in so doing you are keeping your whole body healthy.

*Symptoms*: Painful menstruation, pre-menstrual syndrome (pain, fatigue, irritability), back pain, headache
*Observations*: Unresolved grief, Blood stasis and muscle tension
*Illustrative treatment*: SP4, PC6, GB41, TH5, K7, SP10, LI11, GB20, CV6, ST28, CV12, CV17, Yintang, Trigger points: trapezius, occipitalis, levator scapula, supraspinatus, lumbar paraspinals, quadratus lumborum

**Katya, Age 38**
**Primary Complaint: Migraine**
**Secondary Complaints: Insomnia, Fatigue, Stress**

Katya traveled between the U.S. and Europe on a regular basis for work. Most months she was in Europe for at least one week, and some months she traveled back and forth multiple times. She suffered from migraines, anxiety, and terrible insomnia, which persisted even during her relatively long stays in one city. Her doctor prescribed an anti-anxiety medication, which was the only thing that helped her sleep at night, but as she put it, "I don't want to be on that drug forever."

When she first came to see me, Katya was exhausted. Her pulses showed tiredness throughout her body. Stress and lack of sleep had taken their toll. The paradox about sleep is that you need energy to be able to sleep well. Once you're truly fatigued, that fatigue in itself can prevent good sleep. So this becomes a vicious cycle wherein lack of sleep leads to fatigue, which leads to greater inability to sleep.

I gave her acupuncture to relieve the effects of stress and to activate her body's restorative healing capacity. I used trigger point acupuncture to release the very tight muscles of the upper back and neck, which were contributing to her migraine headaches. Katya slept well after treatment. As she had a rare five-week period without travel, we met twice weekly for treatments to make faster progress. She was sleeping better and better, experiencing much less anxiety, and her migraines were gone.

The big challenge for Katya would be after she returned to frequent traveling. With the stress of her work and travel schedule, along with jet lag (she would often fly all night and start work immediately in the morning without sleep) her lifestyle was likely to drive her back into her symptoms of insomnia and migraines. Most of the people I've seen with frequent work-related travel suffer from the same problems. Katya talked about seeking a new job that would be healthier for her in the long run, but she was not ready yet to take that step.

Katya's experience shows how important it is to adjust your lifestyle to improve your health. If your way of living is continually straining and depleting you, acupuncture isn't going to change that. Sometimes it may seem that you don't have a choice in the matter. Katya seemed to feel this way. It's best to listen to the signs your body is giving you and look for ways to make changes in your life, rather than waiting until your body breaks down completely.

*Symptoms*: Migraines, insomnia, fatigue, stress
*Observations*: Regular international travel interfering with sleep, muscle tension in back, neck and shoulders, multiple systems weak and out of balance
*Illustrative treatment*: K4, PC4, CV17, LI11, LV3, LI4, SP6, ST36, Yintang, Taiyang, GB20, Trigger points: scalenes, sternocleidomastoid, trapezius, supraspinatus, rhomboids, levator scapula, quadratus lumborum, occipitalis

## Erin, Age 30
## Primary Complaint: Migraines
## Secondary Complaint: Neck and Shoulder Pain

Erin suffered from frequent severe migraines. Her headaches were worse before her monthly period. Her mother had a lifelong migraine problem as well, but had found that her migraines let up after menopause. At age 30, Erin didn't want to wait for menopause for relief!

Erin's pulses showed Liver *qi* constraint, a stress-related pattern. The Liver is responsible for the smooth flow of energy in the body. The pain of migraine involves a lack of free flowing energy and so the Liver had be regulated as part of Erin's treatment.

Palpation revealed severe muscle tension in her neck, shoulders and upper back. She worked long hours at the computer, a position that tends to tighten the upper back and neck. As work stress built up, Erin could feel that area getting tighter and tighter.

Erin's treatment focused on restoring free flow through the Liver meridian, while directly releasing the tight muscles in the upper back and neck using trigger point release. After the first treatment, her migraines were relieved. We did a series of eight weekly treatments, getting her through two monthly menstrual cycles, and during this time her

> *Erin's treatment focused on restoring free flow through the Liver meridian, while directly releasing the tight muscles in the upper back and neck using trigger point release. After the first treatment, her migraines were relieved.*

migraines remained at bay and seemed to be gone. Her upper back and neck remained supple and pain-free.

Erin made a conscious effort to mobilize her neck and upper back at work with stretches throughout the day. She also monitored her stress, and when she felt it beginning to settle in the neck area she would take a short break. Erin's part in her own migraine cure was as essential as the acupuncture treatment. By taking an active part, she built on the positive effects of the treatment

*Symptoms*: Migraine headaches, worse before monthly period
*Observations*: Liver *qi* constraint, muscle tension in upper back and neck, physical and emotional stress
*Illustrative treatment*: LV3, PC6, GB41, TH5, SP9, K7, ST36, LI11, Yintang, Trigger points: trapezius, scalenes, temporalis, occipitalis, supraspinatus, levator scapula, rhomboids, quadratus lumborum

## Lora, Age 43
## Primary Complaint: Chronic Bronchitis
## Secondary Complaints: Immune System Weakness, Sciatica, Insomnia, Fatigue, Depression, Allergies

I met Lora when she was 43 years old, married, with a 7-year-old daughter. She was an attorney who had worked almost around-the-clock, seven days a week without a break, even while going through pregnancy, childbirth, and raising her child. She had always enjoyed the challenge of doing it all. She came in for chronic bronchitis, which had been going on for two to three years and had become worse during the previous six months. Lora also complained of reduced energy, insomnia, depression, and sciatica. She suffered from seasonal allergies and several food sensitivities that had recently been diagnosed. As a result she had modified her diet to exclude gluten, dairy, and eggs. She described herself as a very high-energy and positive person suffering from fatigue and depression. Her doctor had prescribed multiple medications including two antidepressants and an anti-asthma drug. She had been on multiple rounds of antibiotics. She wanted to get off the medications. In addition, she was taking a number of supplements including magnesium, zinc, vitamins B12 and D, and probiotics.

Almost 20 years earlier, Lora had appendicitis and had surgery to remove her appendix. Her blood pressure tended to run low and she managed it by adding a little salt to her diet. About two years before coming for acupuncture she had slipped and fallen on ice and had suffered from sciatic pain on her right side since then. Her doctor suspected there might be a problem with her thyroid and she was awaiting those test results. Her mother had died within the last year.

Lora appeared very pale white. Her pulses showed imbalances primarily in the Lungs, Spleen, and Kidneys, with a lot of trapped heat in the Lungs, and pronounced weakness in the Kidneys and immune system. She had a scar on the lower right abdomen from her appendix removal.

Lora presented a complex condition with several interrelated problems that needed to be addressed in tandem for her health to improve. Conventional medicine was giving her medication for the symptoms of bronchial infection, asthma, and depression. Yet she still felt very unwell. Her body needed to be treated as an integrated whole for healing to occur.

In Chinese medicine the Kidneys draw support from the Lungs and the Lungs draw support from the Spleen. Over time, all three of these organ systems had weakened, making her susceptible to digestive and immune system problems as well as bronchitis and asthma. With all of this weakness, her energy flow itself was impaired, so there was an inability for the body to "communicate" internally. To treat her, we needed to strengthen the Kidneys, Lungs, and Spleen while regulating the proper energy flow through the Liver. When there is impaired flow in the Liver, depression often follows. Impaired energy flow that arises out of insufficient energy is like a dried-up stream where water pools instead of rushing downstream as it would if the water were abundant. Depression is just like those pools of water—stagnant energy that does not flow. It feels heavy, and there is no movement.

I treated the patterns of imbalance using acupuncture points on the arms, legs, and back. Lora was amazed to feel the tight, painful muscle on her right waist relaxing upon insertion of an acupuncture point on her leg. This works because the leg point stimulates movement through meridians that pass through the side and back, where the appendix infection and surgery had left an unresolved physical trauma and scar. When there is surgery, the meridian system is disturbed. The body is sewn up but the meridian flow can remain impeded. As a result, that area tends to become weakened. By restoring energy flow through the affected tissue, tension is immediately relieved and the related organ systems are, in a sense, reconnected to the rest of the body. Lora's sciatic pain was on the same side of her body as the surgery. I treated muscles along the pathway of the sciatic nerve to relieve the pain.

I left Lora to rest, and when I returned to the room her facial color had visibly changed and become much less pale. Restored physical vitality was apparent. She opened her eyes and said, "At some point I felt as though I was breathing white." She said she knew that sounded strange but didn't know how else to explain it. I told her it made sense to me and explained, "In acupuncture each organ system has an associated healing color, and the color white is associated with the Lungs." As her Lungs were receiving healing energy from her own body in response to the acupuncture, Lora spontaneously became aware of the healing color flowing in her Lungs.

In traditional acupuncture healing, one can visualize a color to help heal a certain organ system, using the breath to imagine the color flowing through the body, or one can wear that color as another way to help heal the organ system. This may sound implausible, but if you just think about it you'll recognize that when you walk into a room the color of that room can affect your mood and energy level. It's why bars are often painted red and hospitals use muted colors and pastels. According to acupuncture, our color preferences often reveal which of our organ systems need healing and balancing. The ancient acupuncturists didn't write down the process of discovering it; they only wrote down the colors associated with different systems in the body. We don't know how they discovered the locations of acupuncture points and meridians, or what colors heal which organ systems, or how to read the pulses. But Lora's experience gives a glimpse into how they may have made some of these discoveries, through personal experiences like this that occurred within themselves or in patients.

Week by week Lora's energy became stronger and her bronchitis cleared up. As she recovered, she was walking a delicate line. She would experiment with more activity, but if she went a bit too far and did too much, she would suffer a setback and have to rest for several days. This is to be expected in this type of recovery from a deep and chronic illness.

As Lora continued to improve, the setbacks occurred less frequently and required less rest time to recover. I advised her that she would probably have to remain extremely aware of her use of energy over the next couple of years and encouraged her to continue using acupuncture. She agreed that it was time to change her lifestyle, to trim back her work hours, and build in time for rest, relaxation, and time with her family. Many components had contributed to Lora's severe illness. If she had only received acupuncture without making fundamental changes to her life, the results would have been limited. Because Lora took this as an opportunity to make appropriate lifestyle changes, and engaged in her recovery with just as much finesse and enthusiasm as she had brought to her job, she created balance and the opportunity for lasting good health.

*Symptoms*: Cough, upper respiratory allergies, repeated infections, insomnia, fatigue, depression, sciatica
*Observations*: Pale complexion, Lung heat, weak Spleen and Kidneys, constrained Liver *qi*, weak immune system, tight muscles in right lower back, pelvis and leg
*Illustrative treatment*: LU5, LU8, LI4, "Immune points," ST36, K7, LV3, CV6, CV12, CV17, Yintang, abdominal scar tissue, Tight, tender points (right side): biceps femoris, vastus lateralis, gastrocnemius, quadratus lumborum, gluteus medius, piriformis

## Claudia, Age 44
## Primary Complaint: Neck Pain
## Secondary Complaints: Fatigue, Hot Flashes, Insomnia

Claudia came in with severe neck and back pain on the left side. The pain was so bad that it woke her up at night. As a result, she was extremely fatigued. She found herself prone to anger and had a short fuse. She had also begun to suffer from hot flashes, though her period was still regular.

Claudia's pulses and other signs revealed that she was very weakened and tired. Muscle spasms frequently arise out of deep depletion. In her exhausted state, Claudia's body was not strong enough to support healthy structural balance, and her neck pain was an expression of this. If we were to treat only the tension in the neck, the results would be limited and probably short-lived. Strengthening the internal energy was essential to effectively treat Claudia's neck pain.

I used trigger point release to ease the muscle spasms of the neck and back. Other points were selected to help restore strength and to release constrained Liver *qi* which contributed to the pain and led to her excessive anger.

Claudia hoped to return to the gym where she was accustomed to doing vigorous aerobic exercise—the one thing that helped her mood. The problem was that with this degree of weakness in her body, vigorous exercise was too much. Exercise would certainly move the Liver *qi* and relieve her anger and give her a temporary sense of energy, but if too strenuous it would also further exhaust her. She didn't have the inner strength to support it. Claudia needed to start with moderate forms of exercise and gradually work her way up as her strength increased.

Modifying the exercise regimen is often a tough recommendation for people to accept. When the gym routine is the only activity that makes you feel better, you may feel desperate to maintain it. I explained to Claudia that what she really needed was restorative yoga, walking, or even tai chi, which moves the energy and serves as a meditation practice as well. If she did go to the gym, I suggested that she reduce the intensity of her workout: switch to a lower impact exercise and a shorter aerobic workout, then add some stretching. She seemed willing to give it a try.

*After her initial acupuncture treatment, Claudia's neck pain was so much better that she was sleeping well through the night. Within a few treatments over several weeks, her energy and mood were better, her anger was greatly reduced, and the hot flashes were gone too.*

After her initial acupuncture treatment, Claudia's neck pain was so much better that she was sleeping well through the night. Within a few treatments over several weeks, her energy and mood were better, her anger was greatly reduced, and the hot flashes were gone too. She was following the exercise recommendations by reducing the intensity of her workouts and adding some yoga. She was learning to recognize the level of exercise she needed at any given time and to listen to her body's needs.

Once her main complaints had been resolved, Claudia decided to continue using acupuncture to further restore her body. She understood that becoming symptom-free was just the first step and that she had the potential to generate greater strength and balance going forward, especially as she moved through the hormonal changes of perimenopause. Our treatments, which started out twice weekly, then weekly, were eventually scheduled once a month. The key to knowing how frequently to schedule treatments is to note how well the body holds its balance between sessions. Claudia was maintaining well with a monthly treatment. If stress increased or any other symptoms were to arise, even a cold, she knew she could come in sooner for treatment, and we could adjust our schedule as needed to restore balance.

*Symptoms*: Severe neck pain, insomnia, hot flashes, anger, fatigue
*Observations*: Internal depletion, Liver *qi* constraint, adrenal exhaustion, muscle spasms of neck and shoulders
*Illustrative treatment*: K6, LU7, BL62, SI3, ST36, LV4, LV8, LI11, Yintang, BL23, BL14, Trigger points: upper trapezius, splenius cervicis, splenius capitis, supraspinatus, levator scapula

## Margaret, Age 72
## Primary Complaint: Hip Pain
## Secondary Complaint: Herniated Lumbar Disc, Asthma, Weight Gain, Knee Pain

Margaret limped in complaining of severe pain in her right hip. She couldn't sit comfortably or bend down and it hurt all the time. Pain radiated along the back of her leg. She was about 50 pounds overweight and commented that her excess weight was no doubt putting extra pressure on all her joints and that even her knees hurt. She said she had been diagnosed with a herniated disc in her lower back and assumed that her hip and leg pain was coming from there.

When I examined her back, she reported no tenderness around the lumbar discs. There were tight muscles in the buttocks and around the hip joint itself and these were painful to the touch. Because her hip pain was so severe, I went right to work on it by releasing the tight tender points wherever I found them, using trigger point acupuncture. I also used acupoints adjacent to the lumbar spine to help clear inflammation and muscle tension from the lower back, and to relieve stress on the discs. As I touched each painful spot, Margaret exclaimed: "There it is!" She let me know which ones were more sensitive than others and she was gaining confidence that I was on the right track.

As the treatment progressed Margaret began to ask if I could help her with her asthma and weight gain. She had heard about people getting acupuncture for weight loss. I explained that both conditions respond to acupuncture treatment but at the same time she would have to make healthy food choices.

I explained to Margaret a bit more about how acupuncture helps with weight loss, by supporting the digestion, metabolism, nervous system, and healthy function of all the organ systems. If the thyroid function is low, which is sometimes the case when there is weight gain, acupuncture can help it. Usually the adrenal glands, whose job it is to respond to stress, also need to be strengthened. When they are constantly responding to stress of one kind or another, the adrenals secrete excess cortisol, which keeps you from losing weight. In Margaret's case her asthma also reflected adrenal stress. When the Lungs are stressed, as in asthma, the Spleen will also be weakened, which translates into impaired digestion and metabolism. Though it may seem paradoxical, weak digestion promotes weight gain because the body can't properly utilize nutrients. Impaired nourishment to the organs and cells disrupts metabolism and other essential physiological processes. Strong digestion is essential for healthy weight loss. Acupuncture can also reduce food cravings and balance fluctuating blood sugar levels that contribute to them. All of this, together with healthy diet and exercise, serves to promote weight loss.

Margaret returned about a month later to continue balancing the hip, which had remained much better after just one treatment. At that time she mentioned that her right knee bothered her a lot, making it difficult to go up and down stairs. She had had surgery on that knee to repair a torn meniscus a few years ago. When I palpated the knee I could feel taut tissue on the inside of the knee and along the inner thigh. The places where I found these tight spots were where Margaret reported feeling pain. I released these areas by needling them directly until the tissue felt soft and supple. When she got up from the treatment table, Margaret found for the first time in years she was able to walk down the stairs without limping and holding the handrail, and without any pain.

*Symptoms*: Hip pain, knee pain, asthma, weight gain
*Observations*: Spleen and Kidney deficiency, Lung deficiency with heat, structural imbalance, spasms in muscles of hip, pelvis and thigh
*Illustrative treatment*: BL23, BL20, BL18, BL13, Vertebral points adjacent to the lumbar spine, "knee eyes," Trigger points: gluteus medius, piriformis, vastus lateralis, vastus medialis, ileotibial band

## Irene, Age 78
## Primary Complaint: Facial Twitching
## Secondary Complaints: Fatigue, Stress, Depression

Irene had remained active as she aged and walked every day. Walking had also had helped relieve age-related pain in her joints. Seemingly out of the blue, however, she had developed an annoying twitch on the right side of her face, which is what brought her in to try acupuncture. Her doctors hadn't found any obvious reason for the twitching or provided any treatment options.

When I examined Irene, her pulses and other signs revealed a deep exhaustion. Her husband had gone through a prolonged illness and had died within the past year. Irene had always forged ahead in her life whether she was tired or not, so it seemed normal for her to carry on in the face of fatigue. She didn't describe herself as tired or depressed, although I saw clear signs of both. In addition, the muscles in her neck were extremely tight and felt like a rock wall when palpated.

Based on my observations and her history, Irene's facial twitching made sense. Physical exhaustion and stress, coupled with muscle tension in the neck, would provide the ideal conditions for facial twitching to arise as a symptom. In acupuncture terms, she was deficient in *qi* and Blood, and suffered from Liver wind, which showed up as twitching. Her tight neck muscles were probably reducing circulation and pressing on nerves to the face. Caring for her ailing husband and then grieving his death had left her completely drained. Her adrenals had kept her going just long enough to get through it, but once he was gone the depletion hit her and the symptoms started.

Irene's treatment involved boosting her overall *qi* and strengthening the Blood, nourishing the Liver and extinguishing wind, while relieving constrained muscles in the neck using trigger point acupuncture. Because of her deep exhaustion and age, it took about five weekly treatments for the twitch to subside completely. As the twitching resolved, Irene also experienced more energy and a more positive mood.

*Symptoms*: Facial twitching
*Observations*: Tight neck muscles, internal fatigue and exhaustion
*Illustrative treatment*: K3, K7, LV3, LI4, LU7, ST36, SP9, GB20, GV20, Neck and facial points: ST6, ST7, GB14, Tai Yang, Yintang, TH 21, cervical vertebral and muscle points, sternocleidomastoid, scalenes

**Regina, Age 83**
**Primary Complaint: Lower Back and Leg Pain, Difficulty Walking**
**Secondary Complaints: Insomnia, Fatigue**

Regina was a retired dancer and music teacher. She had been through two coronary bypass surgeries and two spinal surgeries to repair herniated discs. She suffered from pain in her lower back and legs, and was only able to walk short distances before she had to sit down and rest. Although her body had been through a lot, her spirit was youthful. She wanted to be out going to the theater, and not confined at home because it was too painful to walk. She had seen her doctor and done physical therapy, without much improvement. Now she was trying acupuncture.

Regina's pulses were weak, reflecting tiredness and reduced resilience, commonly found in older patients. The muscles in her lower back, hips, and thighs were very tight, all part of a misalignment that caused her leg pain. To treat Regina, I selected points to build her *qi* and Blood and to invigorate the circulation, focusing on multiple systems in the body, most fundamentally the Kidneys, which weaken with age. Once the needles were inserted her pulses became stronger and more relaxed, and she fell into a light, restorative sleep. Next, I used trigger points to release some of the tight muscles in the legs, back, and hips. Although physical therapy hadn't helped much before, once her body was strengthened and the trigger points released, it was likely to be more effective in helping her regain and maintain a healthy posture. I encouraged Regina to return to physical therapy while continuing with our treatments.

Little by little we coaxed Regina's muscles out of spasm and balanced her posture so that she could walk increasingly longer distances pain-free. Because of her long history as a dancer, the surgeries, and her advanced age, her body responded more slowly than a younger person's would. Yet in a few months' time she felt significant relief and was able to walk longer distances without any pain. She was also sleeping better at night and feeling more energy during the day.

> *Little by little we coaxed Regina's muscles out of spasm and balanced her posture so that she could walk increasingly longer distances pain-free.*

Acupuncture in older people is effective in relieving many unwanted symptoms that arise in an aging body—many of which have no treatment at all in Western medicine. Expectations must be tailored to the individual. It is not a cure-all and won't bring an 80-year-old back to their 40-year-old self, but it can help immensely to relieve muscle tension and pain, including arthritis, reduce fatigue, improve sleep and mood, and help speed recovery from infections while building immunity.

*Symptoms*: Lower back and leg pain, difficulty walking, insomnia, fatigue
*Observations*: Weak Spleen, Kidney and Heart *qi*, Blood stasis, muscle spasms in lower back, hips and thighs
*Illustrative treatment*: BL62, SI3, K7, BL 23, BL20, BL18, BL14, GB20, lumbar vertebral points, tight, tender points in lumbar paraspinals, gluteus medius, piriformis, biceps femoris, vastus medius, vastus lateralis

## Acupuncture for Fertility and Pregnancy

Since ancient times, acupuncture and Chinese herbal medicine have been used to treat women for infertility, during pregnancy, in labor and delivery, and postpartum. Acupuncture is beneficial at each of these stages. A woman's menstrual cycle, with its regular monthly flow, is an indicator of health and balance. When out of balance, the first step in promoting fertility is to regulate the menstrual cycle.

For women who are trying to conceive, acupuncture is a safe, natural, and effective way to balance hormones, regulate the menstrual cycle, and boost fertility. It is also used to treat men with fertility issues.

The best way to promote fertility and prepare for a healthy pregnancy is to begin balancing the body through acupuncture, diet, exercise and lifestyle a full year before the intended pregnancy. Western science and acupuncture both acknowledge that these factors make a significant difference to the constitution and health of the child throughout its life. That said, most women arrive for treatment right at the time they are hoping to conceive, or having already begun medical fertility procedures – and it is still very effective.

> *We often think in terms of becoming pregnant as the goal of fertility treatment, but the health of both parents at the time of conception and the continuing health of the mother during pregnancy are just as important.*

## Using Acupuncture for Fertility: How Does it Work?

Acupuncture promotes the restoration of hormonal balance and removes blockages in the reproductive system. For most women, this is all that's required to promote fertility and achieve pregnancy. It also relieves stress and supports balance amidst the many emotions raised by fertility challenges, helping you move through healing to pregnancy with greater ease.

How do we assess fertility? A woman's menstrual cycle is the most obvious indicator of reproductive health. By regulating the cycle – most of the time – fertility is naturally restored. The monthly cycle involves an ever-moving, intricate dance of hormonal relationships and regulation. Precisely because of its moving nature, it is especially prone to influences that disrupt flow – including stress of all kinds. The kinds of stress that can affect menstruation range from the daily demands of work and home responsibilities to lack of sleep, catching cold, physical injury, or becoming frustrated, sad or angry for any reason. So basically, being human is filled with many kinds of physical and emotional stresses, each of which can easily impact a woman's reproductive cycle.

Each month the uterus fills with blood in preparation for pregnancy. If there is no pregnancy, that blood is released in menstruation. This monthly filling and emptying of blood in the uterus is subject to blockage, which is known as Blood stasis in acupuncture. Because so much blood moves through the reproductive organs every month, even a small obstruction can build up into a big blockage over time, just as a dam in a flowing river obstructs the water's flow. This is one reason why women are more prone than men to conditions of Blood stasis.

Stasis of Blood in a woman's reproductive system can take the form of uterine fibroids, ovarian cysts, endometriosis, heavy or painful periods, clotting and cramping in menstruation, or blocked fallopian tubes. In conventional medicine these conditions are diagnosed and treated differently. In acupuncture, they are all Blood stasis conditions. Accordingly, the treatment principle is to remove obstruction and invigorate the Blood. Along with Blood stasis, each woman will have her own unique set of imbalances to treat, so no two patients are treated identically with acupuncture, even with the same Western medical diagnosis.

In regulating a woman's cycle, acupuncture also treats symptoms that are commonly associated with pre-menstrual syndrome (PMS) and dysmenorrhea (painful periods): irritability, depression, fatigue, digestive distress, back and leg pain, and headache (including migraines). Because PMS and dysmenorrhea are so common, we come to think of them as "normal." It comes as a happy surprise for most women that it is not normal to suffer through these symptoms, and that acupuncture provides a simple way to eliminate them.

## Birth Control Pills

Conventional medicine frequently uses birth control pills as a way to reduce painful periods and regulate the cycle. There are certainly cases where hormonal therapy may be the right choice for a woman with severe menstrual pain or related symptoms. But it doesn't have to be the first line of therapy. By using acupuncture, most women can regulate their cycle and eliminate unwanted symptoms without using pharmaceutical hormones.

When birth control has been used, there comes a time when many women choose to come off the therapy in order to become pregnant. At this point, acupuncture can be used to regulate the cycle and eliminate unwanted menstrual symptoms. This is the same treatment that in turn supports healthy fertility.

For women coming off birth control pills, depending on factors like the condition of the period before the pill was started and how long it has been used, it may take up to several months of acupuncture to help restore the body's natural hormonal cycles to support fertility.

> *When birth control has been used, there comes a time when many women choose to come off the therapy in order to become pregnant. At this point, acupuncture can be used to regulate the cycle and eliminate unwanted menstrual symptoms. This is the same treatment that in turn supports healthy fertility.*

## Timing of Pregnancy

More women are waiting longer to have their first child. Many women in their 20s and 30s, aware that fertility challenges tend to increase over the age of 35, and especially over age 40, are already trying to decide how long it's "safe" to wait before starting a family. Planning like this is a great idea, when possible, so that your chances of conceiving easily and naturally are improved.

Planning is one thing, worrying is another. A lot of perfectly healthy young women begin to unnecessarily anticipate having a struggle over fertility. The fear that something is wrong with your body is best avoided. Your body knows how to do its job and it was born with the innate ability to regulate and heal itself – with the right support. So even if you feel out of balance or have a condition like polycystic ovarian syndrome (PCOS) or other menstrual irregularities, trust that you can restore your balance to become pregnant. If, after trying natural means of balancing, you are still not getting pregnant, advanced medical fertility procedures are available as a next step when needed.

For younger women, there's usually no need to rush into medical fertility procedures. You have time to work with acupuncture, diet and lifestyle regulation to support fertility and pregnancy. Often a relatively short course of treatment will optimize fertility for women in their 20s or early to mid-30s. Each menstrual cycle is an opportunity to strongly move

Blood and *qi* to better regulate the reproductive system. I advise women to give the process at least three months of treatment before looking for results in the form of pregnancy. However, it is not unheard of for younger women to become pregnant within six to eight weeks of starting treatment.

For women 40 and over, more thought needs to go into the timing of medical fertility interventions. While acupuncture and herbal medicine work to improve fertility at all ages, your natural fertility is declining, especially over 40. You might choose to work with a medical fertility specialist sooner in the process if you are beginning your fertility journey at this age. At the very least, it's a good idea to get an evaluation to find out your medical reproductive status. You can work with a fertility specialist to find out your hormonal balance and the condition of your uterus, fallopian tubes and ovaries. I have often seen women become pregnant soon after the doctor checks for blockage in the fallopian tubes. (This is done, when needed, by flushing a liquid dye through the tubes.) Often the test results show no blockage was present. Yet it seems that the fluids moving through the tubes during the test may have removed some small but significant blockages that had been interfering with fertility.

## Polycystic Ovarian Syndrome

Polycystic ovarian syndrome (PCOS) is a common condition that causes fertility problems in women of all ages. This syndrome involves hormonal imbalances, irregular menstruation, and sometimes ovarian cysts that interfere with fertility. The timing of ovulation in PCOS is often so variable that pregnancy can be elusive. Doctors often tell patients with this diagnosis that they will not be able to conceive naturally. Using acupuncture, I have seen many women with PCOS conceive naturally Acupuncture regulates the hormones and promotes more predictable ovulation cycles. Additionally, underlying patterns of blockage associated with PCOS, including ovarian cysts, can be effectively reduced or eliminated. If acupuncture treatment doesn't sufficiently regulate your cycle after several months, adding medical fertility support to your program may

> *Using acupuncture, I have seen many women with PCOS conceive naturally.*

be the next step. This usually starts with basic testing along with monitoring ovulation to support a natural pregnancy. As needed, increased medical intervention may include pharmaceutical hormonal regulation of the cycle, stimulation of egg production and release, intra-uterine insemination (IUI) or in-vitro fertilization (IVF).

## Preparing for Pregnancy with Acupuncture

As you prepare for pregnancy, it's important to keep in mind that conception and birth aren't completely mechanical, biological processes. A whole new human being with its own soul, spirit and destiny is being brought forth into this world. We can prepare and make all the conditions right to invite pregnancy and birth, but ultimately there's a piece of it that we cannot control. If it takes longer than you anticipated for pregnancy to occur, try to trust the timing, knowing that you are doing all that you can to support it.

When using acupuncture to support fertility, I recommend treatments at least twice a month – ideally just prior to ovulation, and again before the period starts. These are two highly influential points in your cycle to create positive changes through acupuncture. If your period is not regular when you start acupuncture, then you begin with a weekly or twice monthly treatment schedule to regulate your cycle.

As you use acupuncture to regulate your menstrual cycle and promote fertility, you can expect your pre-menstrual symptoms to decrease over the course of a few months, the timing to normalize to 28 days, and the flow to be regulated. It's possible to experience heavier bleeding with or without clots for a few cycles if your body is clearing out Blood stasis from the uterus. Once that is cleared, the flow should normalize and the clots should be eliminated. These are all signs of a healthy reproductive system that best supports fertility.

# Acupuncture to Support Medical Fertility Procedures

## Intrauterine Insemination (IUI) and in-Vitro Fertilization (IVF)

In my clinic, women over 40 have usually already consulted their doctor or a fertility specialist to assess their hormonal status and physical condition by the time they come for acupuncture. Many women at this age hasten to begin medical fertility treatments, whether through medications, in vitro fertilization (IVF) or intrauterine insemination (IUI) procedures. For those who choose medical fertility procedures, acupuncture is a natural support to optimize ovulation, implantation and pregnancy.

Just as acupuncture improves fertility without IVF, it can work to support the use of fertility procedures, while relieving stress. When working with IVF cycles, treatments are timed to complement the medical schedule, promoting growth of strong follicles before egg retrieval, and prepare the body for successful implantation when an embryo is transferred.

Women undergoing IVF typically receive weekly acupuncture treatments leading up to it, and then have a treatment before egg retrieval, and one before and after the transfer. Subsequently treatments are given once or twice weekly until their pregnancy is confirmed.

### Kara, Age 36
### Primary Complaint: Unexplained Infertility

When I met Kara, she was the married mother of a 3-year-old daughter who was conceived using IVF. As a teenager, Kara had begun taking birth control pills to manage her painful periods and remained on them for 10 years, until she married. After she stopped taking birth control, Kara's periods never resumed. Still, she and her husband attempted to have a baby. When, after more than a year, they were unsuccessful, Kara consulted a fertility specialist and began to receive treatments to prepare for in-vitro fertilization. During this process, medications were used to hyper-stimulate ovulation. Multiple eggs were then surgically retrieved from the ovaries and fertilized in the laboratory. Several days after fertilization, a single embryo was selected for surgical implantation in the Kara's uterus. The first two attempts were unsuccessful; the third procedure resulted in pregnancy, and Kara gave birth to her baby girl.

After a couple of years, Kara and her husband returned to the fertility specialist in the hope of repeating IVF using a frozen embryo from the previous procedure. After three attempts, she still hadn't become pregnant and was deeply discouraged. At 36 years of age, the prospect of having a second child seemed to be eluding her.

When I evaluated Kara and heard her history, I was struck by the fact that her periods had never resumed after going off the birth control pill. From my perspective, that would have been the ideal time to use acupuncture to help restore her body's natural cycle. Instead, her doctors jumped straight to using IVF procedures to circumvent her lack of menstruation. Because she had become pregnant, this told us that her eggs and her uterus were healthy, her husband's sperm was healthy, and her body was capable of carrying a pregnancy. Examining Kara, I found a lot of *qi* stagnation and Blood stasis—a lack of proper flow that in women's bodies often impedes menstruation and fertility. Even the fact that Kara had such painful periods as a teenager points to Blood stasis going back at least to that time, a problem that was not resolved but simply suppressed. By the time we met, her reproductive system was "all jammed up" and not functioning well. Through long-term use of birth control hormones, followed by hyper-stimulation during the in-vitro process, her own hormones had been overridden and had failed to resume their proper function.

> *When I evaluated Kara and heard her history, I was struck by the fact that her periods had never resumed after going off the birth control pill.*

Palpation of her lower abdomen revealed quite a lot of tight, tender points and pain. Since the age of 20, Kara had been diagnosed with fibromyalgia and had been in a lot of pain. Here again, acupuncture would see this in broad terms as blockage of flow. The diagnosis of "fibromyalgia" is really no diagnosis at all; it simply reiterates in Latin what you are saying to the doctor, that you have pain in your muscles and fascia. Western medicine gives it a name and sometimes treats its symptoms with medications but doesn't know its origins or how to cure it. Acupuncture sees it in terms of constrained *qi*, usually combined with Spleen and possibly Kidney *qi* deficiency, possible Blood stasis, and inflammation, or deficiency heat. Based on these patterns, acupuncture treats it, often very effectively.

Kara had developed benign nodules on her thyroid gland, which were being monitored. She had also learned that she was gluten-intolerant through medical testing. The gluten intolerance was significant, and she needed to eliminate it from her diet or her body would be perpetually triggered into unwanted immune reactions and inflammation. It is possible that her intolerance to gluten, and possibly to other foods, had created a lot of the inflammation, stasis, and even the thyroid nodules. Or, the reverse: perhaps having the blockage in her body was creating the intolerance to these foods, which, once the blockage was removed, would no longer be problematic for her.

Kara eliminated gluten from her diet and went on a one-month cleansing dietary program to remove potentially allergenic foods and relieve her body's reaction to them. Within two weeks she started to feel more energy than she'd had in years, and her skin was glowing. She was no longer puffy and bloated and had none of the digestive discomfort she'd previously experienced. During this time, she came in for weekly treatments aimed at "waking up" her pituitary and overall endocrine function, strengthening the digestion, moving the Blood and *qi*, and relieving constraint throughout the body. Within weeks her abdomen became soft and supple, without any of the tight, tender spots or palpable masses that we had felt just weeks earlier. For the first time in years she began to feel premenstrual cramping in her lower abdomen. Healthy vaginal mucus reappeared for the first time in years, and her libido returned. After a couple more weeks, Kara got her period for the first time in more than fifteen years.

*The next month Kara cycled again, with noticeable changes mid-cycle but not as intense as the first month, and again she got her period on schedule from then on. After a year of normal, regular cycles, Kara became pregnant naturally.*

The next month Kara cycled again, with noticeable changes mid-cycle but not as intense as the first month, and again she got her period on schedule from then on. After a year of normal, regular cycles, Kara became pregnant naturally.

*Symptoms*: Inability to conceive, amenorrhea (absence of periods), neck and upper back pain, digestive pain and irritability, fatigue, medically diagnosed fibromyalgia, gluten intolerance and thyroid nodules

*Observations*: weak Spleen and Kidney *qi*, Immune weakness, deficiency heat, *qi* constraint, Blood stasis

*Illustrative treatment*: LV3, LI4, LU7, SP9, K7, ST36, "Immune points," ST25, ST28, CV6, CV12, GB20, GB21, moxibustion

## Juliet, Age 28
### Primary Complaint: Chronic Sinusitis
### Secondary Complaint: Polycystic Ovarian Syndrome, Anticipated Infertility Issues

This is a story of how infertility was averted in a patient who came, initially, for acupuncture to treat her sinus congestion. When she first came in, Juliet was suffering from chronic sinusitis. No amount of antibiotics or other medication had helped. After several acupuncture treatments her sinuses had cleared, she had more energy, and she was amazed. Juliet continued to receive acupuncture with some regularity to support her sinus recovery and overall health. Her periods, which had been very long and irregular, generally coming after thirty-five to forty-two days instead of the expected twenty-eight days, began to normalize, and this amazed her as well.

Based on what I observed in Juliet's body signs and pulses, combined with her history of irregular menstruation, I suspected she might be suffering from polycystic ovarian syndrome (PCOS). Acupuncture treats this, usually in terms of the Spleen and Kidney systems. Juliet consulted an endocrinologist who confirmed the PCOS diagnosis. Based on her blood tests and her tendency to gain weight, the doctor put her on a medication intended to normalize the blood sugar levels. Once she started that, she began to lose the excess pounds and had no trouble maintaining her healthy weight.

Over the next two years, as Juliet continued to receive acupuncture, she married and began talking about having a child. Her gynecologist advised that because of her PCOS she and her husband would need to use IVF for pregnancy, and suggested she come in to begin the procedure the following month. The main problem with fertility in PCOS is that ovulation is unpredictable and therefore pregnancy can be elusive. Because Juliet had been receiving acupuncture treatments, which had regulated her menstruation to a twenty-eight day cycle, she became pregnant naturally, and amazed her doctor with the news before the IVF ever got started. A year and a half later she again became pregnant with her second child, also naturally.

There are times with PCOS when IVF is a good way to go, especially if acupuncture hasn't been used or hasn't regulated the menstrual cycle, but Juliet's case illustrates acupuncture's ability to bring a PCOS patient into a normal cycle so that pregnancy can occur naturally.

*Symptoms*: Chronic sinus congestion and infection, allergies, weight gain, irregular menstruation
*Observations*: Spleen and Kidney deficiency, PCOS-like presentation followed by medical diagnosis, immune system weakness, Liver *qi* constraint
*Illustrative treatment*: LV3, PC6, "Immune points," SP9, ST36, K7, CV6, CV12, ST28, GB20, Bi tang, Yintang, moxibustion

## Melinda, Age 32
## Primary Complaint: Migraines
## Secondary Complaint: Inability to Conceive

Melinda's migraines occurred several times a week. They became unbearable every month around the time of her period, and sometimes were so severe that she needed to miss work and spend one or two days in a dark room at home. She mentioned that she was also concerned about fertility. She and her husband had been trying to conceive for the past year and a half, with no luck. After we treated her migraines she wanted to see if there was anything we could do for her fertility. She hadn't yet taken any medical fertility tests, but that would be the next step.

Because migraines are related to a pattern of blocked energy in the body, treatment is aimed at relieving blockage and restoring flow. Menstrual irregularity and pain are also related to a lack of smooth flow in the body. There is frequently a condition of Blood stasis in the reproductive system as a result of impaired energy regulation. Blood stasis can be present even when medical tests show unobstructed fallopian tubes and healthy ovaries and uterus.

When it comes to women's fertility, Blood stasis is one of the very first things we look for, particularly when a woman is young and otherwise healthy. Even in older women there is often a pattern of Blood stasis that is isn't detected by standard medical tests. When this stasis is resolved, pregnancy frequently occurs soon after, within several months of starting acupuncture treatment.

> *When it comes to women's fertility, Blood stasis is one of the very first things we look for, particularly when a woman is young and otherwise healthy. Even in older women there is often a pattern of Blood stasis that is isn't detected by standard medical tests.*

Melinda was delighted with her acupuncture results, as the migraines subsided immediately and she got through that first month's period without having to stay home. She came for treatment weekly. At the end of the second month, her migraines were gone and she was pregnant! In just her second ovulation cycle after we began treating the flow of energy and Blood in her body, Melinda became pregnant naturally. She went on to give birth to a healthy baby girl.

*Symptoms*: Severe migraines several times per week, worse before menstruation, inability to conceive

*Observations*: Liver *qi* constraint with muscle tension in the upper back, neck, and head, Blood stasis with inability to conceive, worsened migraines before the period

*Illustrative treatment*: LV3, PC6, GB41, TH5, SP8, SP10, ST28, GB27, CV6, LI11, Yintang, Taiyang, Trigger points: trapezius, supraspinatus, rhomboids, levator scapula, scalenes, occipitalis, temporalis, quadratus lumborum

**Alison, Age 31**
**Primary Complaint: Fatigue**
**Secondary Complaints: Muscle Pain, Thyroid Imbalance, Infertility**

Alison hadn't come in for fertility treatment. She and her husband wanted to have children but in seven years of marriage there had been no pregnancy. They had discussed adoption. Her main complaint was severe muscle tension and pain throughout the back of her body, from her neck to her ankles. She was also very fatigued, even though she slept deeply and long every night. Her doctor suspected she may have a thyroid problem and when tested, it was shown to be under-functioning.

Alison had been medically diagnosed with hypothyroidism and given thyroid hormone replacement therapy to treat it. She had just begun the medication when she came to see me. She was encouraged that the doctor had found the thyroid problem, as no other doctor had even tested her before, although she had complained of fatigue for years. Probably because Alison was young and didn't exhibit classic signs of hypothyroidism—cold hands and feet, hair loss, weight gain, depression—her previous doctors hadn't considered it.

Another common issue that patients face is that thyroid test results are often misleading. Women who need treatment are sometimes told they are within normal range and are fine. Some doctors are aware that the so-called "normal" ranges are not normal for everyone. These doctors may use a more sensitive test for thyroid function, and others will at least provide the treatment if symptoms suggest that a woman is suffering from hypothyroidism, even if her test results appear in the normal range. The doctor then assesses how the patient responds to treatment. Improvement of symptoms without unwanted side effects generally indicates that the patient has been suffering from a hypothyroid condition.

Low thyroid function is associated with myriad symptoms in the body and may have contributed to Alison's muscle tension as well as to her infertility and fatigue. I expected that as her thyroid improved, her muscles would also relax, her fatigue would lift, and yes—she might also become pregnant.

Could Alison's thyroid condition have been treated with acupuncture alone? Possibly. In her case, because she had begun medical hormone treatment prior to acupuncture, we wouldn't be able to determine this. In some but not all people acupuncture treatment has proven sufficient to restore balance to the thyroid function. Some cases of hypothyroidism are caused by an autoimmune condition known as Hashimoto's thyroiditis. Though it is treated the same way in conventional medicine, in acupuncture it is diagnosed and treated as a different pattern of imbalance.

Once Alison was being medically treated for her hypothyroid condition, acupuncture treatments provided support by strengthening her Kidney *qi* and balancing all her body's systems. I worked directly to relieve muscle tension throughout her back, while focusing on patterns underlying what may have been her infertility (we didn't know whether her husband's fertility was an issue because he hadn't been tested).

> *After six months of acupuncture, while researching adoption options, Alison became pregnant naturally and gave birth to a healthy baby boy.*

Over the course of the next few months, Alison's energy improved, her fatigue was gone, and so were her muscle pains. After six months of acupuncture, while researching adoption options, Alison became pregnant naturally and gave birth to a healthy baby boy.

*Symptoms*: Fatigue, muscle pain, infertility
*Observations*: Medically diagnosed hypothyroidism, weak Spleen and Kidney *qi* with cold, muscle spasms in the lower to upper back
*Illustrative treatment*: K3, K7, SP9, ST36, LV8, LI15, GV20, BL60, BL58, BL40, BL10, moxibustion; Tight, tender points in paraspinal muscles, quadratus lumborum

## Rose, Age 47
## Primary Complaint: Habitual Miscarriage
Rose came for treatment during her first month of pregnancy, which had occurred naturally. She had a five-year-old daughter. In the intervening years, Rose had become pregnant four other times, all of which resulted in miscarriage. This was her fifth pregnancy since having her first child and she desperately wanted to carry it to term.

Miscarriage can of course occur due to abnormalities in the embryo, and that may be a more likely possibility with age. However, when I examined Rose I found a pattern in her body that could explain her inability to hold a pregnancy. In acupuncture it is known as sinking Spleen *qi*, and the remedy is to boost the *qi* using points on the arms, legs, top of the head, and some points on the abdomen or back. After three weekly treatments Rose's pulses and body signs showed a resolution of the pattern. Once that system became strong, as long as the embryo was healthy, I felt that Rose was going to hold this pregnancy, and that's exactly what happened. She continued to come in for treatment throughout her pregnancy and gave birth to a healthy baby girl.

*Symptoms*: Habitual miscarriage (4 times in 3 years)
*Observations*: 1 month pregnant, sinking Spleen *qi*, weak Kidney *qi*
*Illustrative treatment*: GV20, SP9, K3, K7, CV12, PC6, LI11, Yintang

## How Does Acupuncture Help Fertility?[2]

- Research suggests that acupuncture improves the function of the ovaries to produce higher-quality eggs.
- Blood flow to the uterus and ovaries is regulated and strengthened.
- Increased blood flow to the uterus in turn creates a thicker uterine lining. The result is a higher likelihood that the embryo will be implanted in the uterus.
- During implantation of the embryo, it can help avoid uterine contractions, preventing painful cramps and helping to secure the pregnancy.
- Acupuncture can reduce the side effects of the drugs used in IVF, such as emotional instability, insomnia, fatigue, and palpitations.
- For males, acupuncture can improve the quality and quantity of the semen to improve fertility and create better quality embryos.
- Once the patient is pregnant, acupuncture can help to decrease the chances of miscarriage and improve the health of the mother during pregnancy. This translates into improved health of the developing fetus.

# Acupuncture in Pregnancy, Labor and Delivery

I'm often asked if acupuncture is safe during pregnancy. It is more than safe. Most women continue treatments as the pregnancy progresses. During pregnancy, acupuncture helps relieve commonly experienced symptoms.

There are certain acupoints that are traditionally avoided during pregnancy, especially during the first trimester, but even those may be used in some cases, when the patient's individual condition indicates it. It would be extremely difficult to interrupt a healthy pregnancy with acupuncture. However, not all pregnancies start off strong. In an abundance of caution we emphasize points that help secure pregnancy and avoid those whose function is known to draw the body's energy downwards.

The first trimester commonly brings nausea and fatigue. There can be other digestive complaints, including heartburn, as well as lower back or neck pain. All of these can be treated using acupuncture.

The second trimester tends to be the most symptom-free. The nausea and fatigue of the first trimester have typically subsided. Common complaints include heartburn, constipation, varicose veins, hemorrhoids, and backache or sciatica, all of which can respond favorably to acupuncture.

As the pregnancy progresses to the third trimester women often experience more physical discomfort due to the excess weight and strain on the back and legs. There may be difficulty finding comfortable a position, especially to sleep. Insomnia and anxiety may occur or increase. Back and leg pain, sciatica, carpal tunnel syndrome and swelling are common complaints at this stage.

Before going into labor, acupuncture and moxibustion can also help turn a breech baby. At the right time, it can also be used to help induce and facilitate labor itself.

During all stages of pregnancy, many women seek out acupuncture to treat conditions for which they might have used medications prior to pregnancy. This includes immune system support, treatment for hay fever and other allergy symptoms, colds, headache, insomnia, and mild urinary tract infections.

Babies in the womb seem to love acupuncture. As soon as the mother's acupuncture points are stimulated, she commonly feels the baby moving more actively. This makes sense as the baby's whole environment is the mother's body, so as energy moves and changes in response to acupuncture treatment, the baby will naturally feel it too. Hopefully the baby will settle down after the initial movement so the mother can get a much needed rest during her acupuncture session!

## Before Delivery: Treatment of Breech Presentation

If the fetus remains in breech position after thirty-four weeks, obstetricians often send their patients to an acupuncturist, specifically for treatment with moxibustion (a warming herb), as way of turning the baby. There is an empirical point (BL67), observed to work clinically, located on the little toe, which stimulates the baby to turn. Movement may occur after one treatment or it may take several treatments. The patient can be taught to continue self-treatment at home, with help from her partner. However, the midwife or obstetrician must monitor the baby's position so that it doesn't turn back into breech position in response to ongoing treatment.

## Labor and Delivery

In healthy pregnancies acupuncture can be used to support labor and to help induce it naturally at full term or when the due date has passed. This is done with the approval of the physician or midwife and is not used for this purpose when medical preconditions exist.

The same points that are avoided in early pregnancy to avoid disrupting it are now used, with intense stimulation, to help induce labor. Treatments can be given daily until the onset of labor. In my experience acupuncture helps to initiate contractions, often within several hours.

Acupuncture can be given during labor to relieve pain and anxiety, reduce the duration of labor, and facilitate delivery. During later stages of labor and delivery, the ear points are usually selected for treatment because of the physical movement involved in the birthing process, although other points may be used as well.

## Postpartum

Once the baby is born, everyone's focus tends to shift to the baby's needs, and the mother's recovery is almost completely ignored or left to chance. However, this is an incredibly important time to care for the mother. Having been through pregnancy, labor, and delivery, she needs to restore her physical and emotional well being. Her *qi* and Blood have been depleted by labor and delivery. Typically, she is exhausted. She begins to breastfeed the baby while usually getting just a few hours of broken sleep each night.

In China it is still part of the culture to take care of the mother after childbirth. With this awareness, the new mother and her baby stay home for the first 40 days. During this time a family member or a special caretaker will cook nutritious, healthy food for the mother, provide her with herbal remedies to build her up, and help look after the baby so the mother can rest. Contrast this with our own culture in which the parents are often on their own to care for the newborn. The mother gets little rest or sleep. Within days or weeks she often wraps the baby up and goes out to shop or meet people or take care of other responsibilities. Meanwhile, who has taught the parents how to care for a newborn? They're learning on the job. Every rash, every cry, every symptom is a new unknown challenge. Sometimes a grandmother will come to stay and help out, but it's been so long since she had her own babies that she herself doesn't really remember how to do it! And there is still very little attention to nurturing the mother's health at this time.

*During this time a family member or a special caretaker will cook nutritious, healthy food for the mother, provide her with herbal remedies to build her up, and help look after the baby so the mother can rest.*

We may not be able to have a fulltime caretaker come and stay with us, but there's a lot more we can do to restore a mother's health after childbirth. You can help rebuild *qi* and Blood through acupuncture, moxibustion, nutrition and herbal remedies. This will build strength, which in turn supports healthy lactation for breastfeeding. Acupuncture also builds immunity, which is often compromised when *qi* and Blood are depleted. Significantly, this will help rebalance hormone levels and regulate mood to avert or alleviate depression—a major, sometimes severe, postpartum challenge for many women.

## Acupuncture for Men's Health

"Man up, guys. You're not going to let a bunch of tiny
needles keep you from being your best are you?!"
- Fred Schuster

Men's health challenges commonly treated with acupuncture include pain syndromes, sports injuries, low sex drive and impotence, prostatitis, prostate enlargement and frequent or difficult urination, snoring, allergies, gout, acid reflux, insomnia, weight gain, diabetes and high blood pressure, among others.

A challenge for men in our culture is being taught that masculinity entails never showing weakness or vulnerability. As a result, men often wait too long before seeking treatment. In particular a lot of men are hesitant to try acupuncture for problems other than pain. It is frequently a wife, girlfriend, mother or daughter that gets a man in for treatment with acupuncture. Sharing men's stories of healing through acupuncture for a variety of conditions may help others to see how it might benefit them as well.

## Men's Healing Stories

**Adam, age 42**
**Primary Complaint: Acid Reflux**
**Secondary Complaints: Low Sex Drive, Insomnia, Anxiety, Stress**
Adam suffered from persistent acid reflux and had been diagnosed with precancerous cells in the esophagus. He also complained of a low sex drive, stress, anxiety, and insomnia.

Adam had been prescribed antacids, which he took regularly, but the reflux still broke through, and he wanted to get off the medications. When he came to me he had recently modified his diet and informed his doctor that he was experimenting with not using the medication. He was aware that eating certain foods made the reflux worse, as did eating late at night.

Evaluation revealed underlying weakness in the digestive system, and stress causing blocked energy flow and circulation. In the language of acupuncture, he exhibited a pattern of heat rising from the Stomach that can lead to injury to the Heart. Although conventional medical tests would most likely not find any heart problems, he was a clear candidate for future heart disease if something wasn't done.

Because conventional medicine has no test to support this diagnosis, his doctors would likely tell him his heart is fine, and that the reflux condition has no relationship to the health of his heart. Of course it is not the reflux causing the heart disease, but a pattern of imbalance in the body that can lead to both conditions. When we recognize the integrated nature of the human system, and how patterns of imbalance cause multiple symptoms, we can get to the root cause, practicing restorative and preventive medicine.

Fortunately, Adam was motivated to treat his acid reflux and hoped that acupuncture could also reduce his stress and anxiety, improve his sex drive, and help him sleep. I knew that by balancing the patterns behind these conditions, we would also be balancing those that could lead to heart problems in the future.

After just a few months of treatment two to three times a month, Adam reported increased sex drive, greatly improved sleep, and reduced stress and anxiety. To his amazement, his medical checkup showed that his esophagus had no sign of the precancerous cells that had been there

> *After just a few months of treatment two to three times a month, Adam reported increased sex drive, greatly improved sleep, and reduced stress and anxiety. To his amazement, his medical checkup showed that his esophagus had no sign of the precancerous cells that had been there before.*

before. He achieved this with acupuncture and watching his diet—without using antacid medication. Adam was so convinced of the effectiveness of this approach, and so relieved with this seemingly miraculous recovery, that he chose to continue using acupuncture once or twice monthly to maintain his health gains and continue to improve.

*Symptoms*: Acid reflux, precancerous cells in esophagus, low sex drive, insomnia, anxiety

*Observations*: Red tongue, weak, rapid pulse, signs of Stomach yin deficiency with heat, heat in the Heart, Spleen and Kidney *qi* deficiency

*Illustrative treatment*: K3, SP9, ST36, LV8, LI11, HT3, CV4, CV6, CV12, CV14, Yintang

**Grant, Age 50**
**Primary Complaint: Numbness in Feet**
**Secondary Complaint: Lower Back Pain, Lumbar Disc Herniation**

Grant was a construction worker who suffered from disc herniation in the lumbar spine, causing numbness in both feet when he was standing or sitting for prolonged periods. My initial evaluation showed that Grant had both deficiency and blockage of Blood and *qi*. Treating the numbness in his feet would include strengthening Blood and *qi* and getting it all moving throughout his body.

Grant had quite a bit of muscle tension on both sides of his lumbar spine, which I typically find with disc herniation. The disc is herniated because it has become overly compressed and the muscles in the area are tight. This muscle tension can put pressure on the nerve root as it emerges from the spine, causing pain and numbness down the legs and into the feet. Tight muscles in the back, hip, and leg can also squeeze the nerve along its pathway, adding to the problem. In addition, there may be inflammation at the site of the herniated disc, which causes its own pain. In Grant's case, he didn't currently have inflammation or pain at the disc itself.

I released the muscle tension in his lower back to create freedom of movement and space for the spine to elongate. This takes pressure off the disc, relieving pressure on the nerve root. I also treated the muscle spasms that I found in the hip and leg, which were contributing to the structural imbalance and perpetuating the numbness.

The muscular component in this type of pain syndrome is typically not addressed in conventional medicine. My patients who arrive with disc herniation have usually been to the doctor (which is where they receive the diagnosis, usually through an MRI). Often the doctor has prescribed physical therapy, which can do a lot to relieve structural pressure on the disc or the nerve, but may not be enough to completely cure it. Anti-inflammatory medications and muscle relaxants are commonly prescribed. Sometimes, especially with severe pain, cortisone injections are used directly in the affected area to relieve pain and inflammation. This sometimes relieves the acute pain very well, but physical therapy and acupuncture are still recommended to heal the area and avoid a recurrence. At other times up to three shots will be administered, with no noticeable improvement. When all else fails, surgery frequently becomes the next option.

Grant's doctor had talked to him about surgery as a future possibility, while encouraging him to use physical therapy and acupuncture first. The numbness in Grant's feet was more than a matter of discomfort; it made it difficult for him to feel where he was walking, which seriously affected his balance, potentially leading to accidents. As his work involved lifting, climbing, and moving heavy objects, this was a particularly serious risk.

I chose acupuncture points to treat Grant's *qi* and Blood deficiency and blockage. I used additional points around the affected discs, and did trigger point release on the lower back muscles to relax the area and create more space for the nerves to pass unobstructed. His feet were treated directly using points that help relieve neuropathy in the feet, whatever the cause.

While the acupuncture needles were in place, Grant fell into a deep restful sleep for about thirty minutes. When he woke up, he said he felt as if all the acupuncture points were connected by a network of "energy." It was, for him, a very tangible experience of energy working in his body. He felt restored and rested in a way that never happened for him during an ordinary night's sleep.

Over the course of several sessions, the numbness in his feet diminished. Its frequency and intensity were reduced until he barely noticed it at all. He also had more energy and strength, and his sense of well-being had improved. Because his condition was chronic and somewhat advanced, we continued intermittent treatments to support his recovery and improvement.

*Symptoms*: Numbness in the feet, lumbar disc herniation
*Observations*: Tight muscles in the lower back, internal deficiency of *qi* and Blood, Blood stasis and *qi* constraint

*Illustrative treatment*: BL62, SI3, K6, LU7, LV8, ST36, SP9, Bafeng points on the foot, BL23, BL20, BL18, lumbar vertebral points; Trigger points: lumbar paraspinals, quadratus lumborum, piriformis, gluteus medius

## Calvin, Age 45
### Primary Complaint: Bronchitis
### Secondary Complaints: Insomnia, Weak Immune System, Fatigue, Recurrent Bronchitis and Pneumonia

Calvin had severe bronchitis and insomnia when he came for acupuncture. He looked pale, with dark circles under his eyes. He was friendly and animated, with a warm personality. The way he explained it, he knew he needed rest to recover, but he just couldn't quiet his mind enough to fall asleep. The minute he put his head down on the pillow, he began to think, plan, and problem-solve. He also liked the nighttime hours for his creative work, so he didn't keep a regular sleep schedule. He would often stay up into the early hours of the morning making art. Frequently he would wait until he was beyond exhausted to go to bed because it was the only way he could fall asleep. He'd had this problem for as long as he could remember.

His inability to sleep had led to fatigue and weakened immunity, and he had frequent colds. This had progressed to repeated bouts of bronchitis and pneumonia. His doctor had put him on several rounds of antibiotics, but Calvin still had an unrelenting cough and profound fatigue.

After a few acupuncture treatments, Calvin's bronchitis had cleared up. He was sleeping better

> *The key to resolving his bronchitis was not antibiotic treatment, which wasn't working anyway. The bacterial infection only occurred because he had so weakened his lungs and immune system through stress, lack of sleep, and an unregulated schedule. Acupuncture helped him regain strength and balance so that his body could heal itself.*

and feeling more energy during the day. He was coming up with some strategies to reduce his stress and improve his sleep. For example, if he listened to music he was able to fall asleep much earlier in the evening and sleep through the night. He scheduled his work to end earlier in the evening and added daily exercise early in the day.

Calvin continued coming for treatments for several months to continue strengthening his body and immune system and support the positive lifestyle changes he was making to improve his health. The key to resolving his bronchitis was not antibiotic treatment, which wasn't working anyway. The bacterial infection only occurred because he had so weakened his lungs and immune system through stress, lack of sleep, and an unregulated schedule. Acupuncture helped him regain strength and balance so that his body could heal itself.

*Symptoms*: Coughing, fatigue, insomnia
*Observations*: Irregular work and sleep schedule with underlying anxiety, weak Lungs, Spleen, Kidneys, immune system weakness
*Illustrative treatment*: LU5, LU7, LI4, "Immune points," K7, LV3, SP9, ST36, Yintang, CV17, CV12, CV6, moxibustion

## Dennis, Age 75
## Primary Complaint: Restless Leg Syndrome
## Secondary Complaint: Lower Back Pain, Sciatica

Dennis was a retired firefighter who had been through a successful triple coronary bypass operation. Since his surgery, several years prior to his first acupuncture visit, he had been exercising and had changed his diet to support his heart health. However, he was suffering from Restless Leg Syndrome (RLS), which kept him awake at night. His legs felt like they needed to be moved all the time, and he couldn't rest. His doctors had tried various medications, none of which had helped. In desperation, he sought out acupuncture as a last hope. Dennis also suffered from lower back pain and occasional sciatic pain down the left leg.

Although Western medicine sees correlations between RLS and other conditions, it doesn't know the cause of it, nor does it have a curative treatment. In acupuncture, RLS is often associated with *qi* deficiency and impaired circulation, and it is treated by rectifying these imbalances. As an older heart patient, it was reasonable to assume that Dennis's circulation was weak. Circulation would be even slower at night while lying down in one position for sleep. Even without RLS, people often complain of lower leg cramps at night, related in part to the reduced circulation in the legs.

In Dennis's case, his pulse and body signs showed weakness in the Heart, Spleen, Liver and Kidneys. Palpation showed tight muscles in the lower back and buttocks, and an imbalance of the pelvis, which together were causing pressure on the left sciatic nerve. I selected acupoints on various meridians to build and invigorate *qi* and Blood, which includes improving digestion and circulation. I also used trigger point release in the lower back and buttocks to relieve tension that was leading to sciatic pain.

After six weekly acupuncture treatments, Dennis's symptoms were completely resolved. He no longer suffered from Restless Leg Syndrome or sciatic pain, and he reported sleeping much better with more energy during the day.

*Symptoms*: "Restless legs" especially at night, interfering with sleep
*Observations*: History of cardiac bypass surgery, weak *qi* and Blood with Blood stasis, tight muscles in the lower back and buttocks
*Illustrative treatment*: ST36, SP9, K7, LV3, LI4, LI11, HT3, Trigger points: lumbar paraspinals, quadratus lumborum, gluteus medius, piriformis

## Danny, Age 32
## Primary Complaint: Restless Leg Syndrome
## Secondary Complaints: Insomnia, Fatigue, Stress

While Restless Leg Syndrome (RLS) is more often seen in older people, Danny was a young man with a severe case of it, and he also had insomnia. He had been working without a break since completing graduate school and had built a successful career, but was still working incessantly. He had recently married and his wife sent him for acupuncture when she realized the severity of his insomnia.

Danny was suffering from adrenal fatigue and a deficiency of *qi* and Blood, among other imbalances. In addition to a series of acupuncture treatments, it was time for him to restructure his work so that he was not perpetually depleting his internal resources. Would he be willing to do this? Many young men in their 30s are still building their careers, putting aside all other considerations. Like Danny, they aren't yet motivated to make the necessary changes.

The acupuncture treatments he received were few and far between as he never found the time to come in, and he didn't make any changes to his busy routine. As a result, he continued to live with his RLS.

Two years passed, and Danny was back in my clinic for treatment. His RLS had become even more severe, and now he was also suffering from anxiety and occasional panic attacks. He and his wife had had their first child. He had hit rock bottom and simply could not go on. Finally, he was motivated to change.

We followed a course of weekly acupuncture treatments along with herbal medicine that he took daily. He decided to make lifestyle changes, including ending work each night by 7 p.m. and relaxing before going to bed at a reasonable hour. By this time he was taking sleep medications prescribed by his doctor, yet he was still only getting four to five hours of sleep a night. I asked him to commit to eight hours of sleep each night, to increase his water intake (he rarely drank water during his busy days), to begin a very gentle exercise regimen, and to eat regular meals in a calm manner. His wife agreed to support this program even though it meant more of the child care fell to her.

*Danny followed the program and within four weeks he was able to sleep without medication. His RLS was nearly gone, though it still woke him up at times. After eight weeks he felt like a new person. He was able to sleep through the night and had clarity and focus that he had long since lost through lack of rest and overwork.*

Danny followed the program and within four weeks he was able to sleep without medication. His RLS was nearly gone, though it still woke him up at times. After eight weeks he felt like a new person. He was able to sleep through the night and had clarity and focus that he had long since lost through lack of rest and overwork. Though he was now working shorter hours (down to a 40-hour workweek from approximately 80 hours) he felt more productive and satisfied than he was before. Like Danny, many people need to get to the breaking point before being willing to change their habits and their lives.

*Symptoms*: "Restless legs," insomnia, fatigue, anxiety, panic attacks
*Observations*: Severely depleted *qi* and Blood affecting Spleen, Stomach, Liver, Heart and Kidneys
*Illustrative treatment*: LV4, LV8, K4, PC4, SP9, ST36, LI11, CV17, Yintang, GB20

## Marcos, Age 35
## Primary Complaint: Sciatica
## Secondary Complaints: Lower back pain, Herniated Lumbar Discs, Seasonal Allergies, Fatigue

Marcos came in complaining of sciatic pain that started at the hip and moved down the back of his leg. He sometimes felt the pain all the way to his outer ankle. He had a history of back pain, and MRIs had shown herniation to the discs at the levels L2, L4, and L5. He had kept it under control through exercise, but in recent months his exercise had lapsed because of long work hours and having a family with two small children.

Sciatica is a very common complaint that is often incorrectly assumed to be a permanent diagnosis. It's usually relatively easy to resolve using acupuncture. The main exception to this is when advanced stenosis of the lumbar spine puts pressure on the sciatic nerve – then it is harder to treat. In most people sciatica is caused mainly by pelvic imbalance and muscle spasms along the pathway of the sciatic nerve, or by a combination of muscle spasms and lumbar disc herniation.

> *Sciatica is a very common complaint that is often incorrectly assumed to be a permanent diagnosis. It's usually relatively easy to resolve using acupuncture.*

In Marcos's case, it was a combination of the two: he had very tight muscles along the spine on both sides, indicating compression of the lumbar spine, slight sensitivity in the lumbar discs, and tight muscles along the pathway of the sciatic nerve, including the gluteals, piriformis, hamstrings, and gastrocnemius.

Marcos was also suffering from seasonal allergies, which had recently worsened, as well as fatigue. Since he had been under more stress for several months, not only had he given up his exercise, but his body's overall resilience had suffered. He displayed signs of deficient Spleen *qi*, which leads to fatigue and immune weakness, constrained Liver *qi*, one of the root causes of pain, and deficient Kidney *qi*, which reduces the body's ability to respond to stress, increases inflammation, lowers immunity, and is associated with lower back weakness and pain.

To treat Marcos's pain, we would have to improve all of these internal systems. If we only treated his back, our success would be limited. Many external "excess" conditions of joint inflammation and muscle spasm have at the root some form of internal "deficiency."

Metaphorically, one way to look at it is if you're weak inside, your outer structures—the muscles—have to hold on tighter to keep you together. When there is support coming from within the body, then the exterior muscles don't need to work as hard. They are also better nourished and can function well, without going into spasm.

In treating Marcos I focused on strengthening his Spleen and Kidney *qi*, and harmonizing the flow of Liver *qi*, while also clearing inflammation. I treated his back adjacent to the lumbar spine to relieve pain and inflammation and used trigger point release on the lumbar paraspinal muscles to relieve compression from the discs. The same method relieved spasms in the muscle groups along the pathway of the sciatic nerve that were compressing the nerve.

Marcos felt significant pain relief after one treatment. It took three treatments to fully restore balance in his back and eliminate the pain. Because he had a disc vulnerability and lived a stressful life, he chose to use acupuncture as a periodic form of preventive care for his back and to eliminate his allergies and other effects of stress on his body.

*Symptoms*: Sciatic pain radiating down the leg, lower back pain, seasonal allergies, fatigue
*Observations*: Overwork, stress, constrained Liver *qi*, weak Spleen and Kidney *qi*, immune system weakness, tight muscles in lower back, hip and leg
*Illustrative treatment*: BL40, BL58, BL60, BL10, BL23, BL20, BL18, BL13, lumbar vertebral points, Trigger points: quadratus lumborum, lumbar paraspinals, gluteus medius, piriformis, biceps femoris, gastrocnemius

## Derek, Age 37
## Primary Complaint: Plantar Fasciitis
## Secondary Complaints: Fatigue, Constipation

Derek was an accountant and married father of two who loved running for exercise and relaxation. He was suffering from plantar fasciitis, an intense pain in his left foot when he walked or ran, which inhibited his ability to do both. It had been bothering him for the past four months, and recently he'd had to stop running altogether.

Plantar fasciitis is a common problem involving inflammation of the fascia, or connective tissue, in the foot. Acupuncture is very effective in treating it. When there is foot pain, there is almost always a structural imbalance further up the leg, into the hip, pelvis, and lower back. This imbalance comes about for many reasons—for example, how you stand, sit, or strain your muscles in exercise. When one part "goes out," the strain or muscle tension is transmitted to other parts of the body, which are now trying to compensate. In runners it's common to find muscle tension extending from the lower back down through the legs and into the feet. Runners pay attention to the quality of running shoe used, and to buying new shoes frequently to support the feet, but the imbalances in muscles above the feet are often overlooked.

> *Plantar fasciitis is a common problem involving inflammation of the fascia, or connective tissue, in the foot. Acupuncture is very effective in treating it. When there is foot pain, there is almost always a structural imbalance further up the leg, into the hip, pelvis, and lower back*

Derek also complained of fatigue and constipation. In addition to structural imbalances from running, his internal condition also contributed to the symptom of plantar fasciitis. Acupuncture treatment included points to strengthen the internal weakness, Spleen *qi* deficiency and dryness that was contributing to his fatigue and constipation.

Plantar fasciitis can occur in different parts of the foot. Derek described having pain in the outer aspect of the left foot and heel, suggesting that he was likely to have muscle tension on the outer leg and into the hip, which is exactly what I found through palpation. In addition to treating the internal imbalances that were revealed through Derek's pulse qualities, I directly released trigger points in the lateral quadriceps of the thigh and peroneal muscles of the lower leg, as well as treating the foot itself.

After a single treatment, Derek's foot pain was gone and he was able to resume running. I suggested methods of stretching and balancing the legs, lower back, and pelvis as a regular practice to avoid the imbalance that brought on the foot pain in the first place and to remain pain-free.

*Symptoms*: Foot pain and inflammation, fatigue, constipation
*Observations*: Qi deficiency and dryness, tight muscles in upper and lower leg, tightness and inflammation of fascia in the foot
*Illustrative treatment*: LV3, LI4, LU7, LI11, ST36, SP6, Yintang, plantar fascia points, K6, BL61, Trigger points: quadriceps, peroneals

## Anthony, Age 38
## Primary Complaint: Seasonal Allergies
## Secondary Complaints: Fatigue, Stress

When I met Anthony he was working long hours as a corporate attorney and was a married father of two young children. He sought treatment for his seasonal allergies, which had worsened over the past couple of years. Through diet and exercise, he had lost 30 pounds over the past year and stayed fit by attending the gym almost daily.

Anthony's pulse and body signs showed very deficient Spleen *qi* and overall exhaustion with an overlay of stress. It is quite typical for the Spleen to become weak in people who lose weight. In the process of losing weight, by definition you are taking in fewer calories than you require on a daily basis, so that your body then draws on its own fat stores for energy. While the Spleen is responsible for generating *qi*, it is also the system most directly affected by calorie restriction and may itself become weakened. Another aspect of the Spleen is related to the lymphatic and immune systems in Western terms. When the Spleen becomes depleted, it begins to affect every other system in the body. When you have a stressful and demanding schedule, as Anthony did, your Kidney *qi* also gets used up. In Western terms this translates into adrenal exhaustion. Now you have a "perfect storm" for the activation of seasonal allergies. The adrenal system isn't able to help your body adapt to stress, and its anti-inflammatory function becomes impaired; the deficient Spleen leads to immune and lymphatic dysfunction and overall energetic depletion; the Liver is both undernourished and strained by stress and so it fails to circulate the "wei *qi*" (protective energy) that translates in part into immune strength in the body.

The treatment for seasonal allergies in a case like Anthony's involves strengthening all the body's systems, starting with the Spleen, Kidneys and Lungs, while regulating the Liver at the same time. I advised him to find ways to get more daily rest and reduce his stress. He was no longer dieting, so he was now eating sufficient daily calories, which helped. In addition to the quantity of food, other ways to strengthen the Spleen include eating easily digestible foods, emphasizing warm and cooked foods over cold and raw foods, staying away from cold drinks, drinking water at room temperature rather than chilled, eating at regular intervals, and stopping work to eat calmly while chewing food thoroughly. There was only so much Anthony could do about his schedule because of his responsibilities, but he did what he could.

After his initial acupuncture treatment Anthony experienced immediate symptomatic relief and his seasonal allergies cleared up completely after five weekly treatments.

*Symptoms*: seasonal allergies, fatigue
*Observations*: Stressful lifestyle, recent weight loss, weak Spleen, Lung and Kidney *qi*, Liver *qi* constraint, immune system weakness
*Illustrative treatment*: K3, K7, LV4, "Immune points," SP9, ST36, LU7, LI4, CV12, Yintang

**Marty, Age 58**
**Primary Complaint: Hip Pain**
**Secondary Complaints: Weight Gain, Insomnia**
Marty was a financial analyst who came for acupuncture with severe hip pain and joint degeneration. The pain seriously limited his daily activities. He was unable to exercise, and even standing and walking were painful. He woke in pain frequently during the night. He was scheduling hip replacement surgery within the next few months.

When the hip joint has degenerated to this degree, surgical hip replacement is virtually the only way to relieve pain and restore function. Structural imbalances that lead to hip degeneration, if treated years earlier, can often be corrected, taking the destructive pressure off the joint, averting injury and the need for later surgery. To do this, we need to be alert to the smaller pains and imbalances that occur along the way and to treat them instead of overlooking them.

> *Structural imbalances that lead to hip degeneration, if treated years earlier, can often be corrected, taking the destructive pressure off the joint, averting injury and the need for later surgery.*

Patients come for acupuncture with hip pain at various stages. Some arrive at a late stage in hope of delaying surgery as long as possible, or like Marty, to get some pain relief while awaiting surgery. Depending on how advanced the degeneration is, acupuncture can often help avoid the need for surgery altogether. If eventual surgery is inevitable, it can provide significant temporary pain relief that buys time before doing the surgery. It also helps to restore structural balance prior to surgery. When a new hip joint is screwed into position, you want your pelvis to be as balanced as possible so the surgery doesn't lock you into the wrong alignment. After surgery, acupuncture can help your recovery, along with physical therapy.

In Marty's case, his hip pain had not only disrupted his sleep, exhausting him, but it prevented him from exercising, and he had gained weight. The surgeon wanted him to lose at least twenty to thirty pounds prior to surgery to make recovery easier, but he was in a bind because the pain prevented exercise and rest, making it very difficult to take off the weight.

Marty wasn't really expecting acupuncture to help, but when he got off the treatment table he was amazed at how much better he felt. He could stand straighter and walk without any pain. By continuing with weekly treatments, Marty was able to resume moderate exercise and sleep soundly while living with much less pain. In addition to following a healthy diet, this allowed him to lose twenty-five pounds over the next few months in advance of his hip replacement surgery.

*Symptoms*: Severe hip pain disrupting sleep, inability to exercise, weight gain
*Observations*: Hip joint tenderness, pain, and inflammation, tight muscles in lower back, pelvis and leg, internal weakness affecting the Spleen, Liver, Kidney and Heart
*Illustrative treatment*: K7, ST36, GB34, SP9, LV3, LI4, PC4, LI11, Yintang, BL23, BL20, BL18, BL14; Trigger points: lumbar paraspinals, quadratus lumborum, gluteus medius, piriformis, biceps femoris, gastrocnemius

## Brian, Age 51
## Primary Complaint: Back Pain
## Secondary Complaints: Diabetes, Weight Gain

Brian came for acupuncture to treat his back pain. He ran his own business as a construction contractor. As a result of his strenuous physical labor, he regularly strained his back, which hurt everywhere. He had been doing this work for years, but he no longer tolerated the physical strain or recovered as quickly as he did when he was younger. Over the last several years he had also gained about 40 pounds of weight and was recently diagnosed with type 2 diabetes. His dietary choices weren't helping – he preferred bread, pasta, cookies and sweets, and meat, but no vegetables, fruits or fresh food of any kind. He was cheerful and enjoyed his work, but he was also physically exhausted. As soon as I put the acupuncture needles in, Brian fell sound asleep.

I treated his back pain by first using points to strengthen his Spleen, with an emphasis on the pancreas, and points to balance the Liver and Kidneys as well. I used points to regulate blood sugar and support the adrenals, which had become weak from stress and exhaustion. Next I treated the muscle groups on both sides of the spine, which were extremely tight and tense. Finally I treated his back with tuina massage to help further relax the muscles and move the *qi*. It wasn't until Brian's third treatment that I began to treat specific muscles with trigger point release. First we had to get the overall tightness in the back to relax with more general restorative points. Once that was done, the remaining tight tender points could be isolated through palpation and treated with trigger point release.

While treating Brian's back pain, I was necessarily strengthening his whole body, including the Spleen and pancreas. I worked with Brian on his food choices because no amount of acupuncture could overcome his diabetes unless he made changes to his diet. He had to start eating whole foods without skipping meals, incorporating healthy, low-glycemic index snacks during the day, and drinking more water. His wife was eager to support him in making these changes and made a special effort to prepare his meals and join the dietary program along with him.

Brian received weekly treatment for 3 months and then tapered to twice monthly and then once a month. In the first 3 months of acupuncture Brian had lost 30 pounds, his back pain had reduced significantly, his blood sugar had normalized, and he was feeling better than he had felt in 20 years. Once he got used to the new diet and felt the benefits it was easier to follow and maintain. When he lapsed, which he did from time to time, he recovered quickly by coming in for more regular treatments to help him get back on his healthy program.

> *In the first 3 months of acupuncture Brian had lost 30 pounds, his back pain had reduced significantly, his blood sugar had normalized, and he was feeling better than he had felt in 20 years.*

*Symptoms*: Back pain, weight gain, type 2 diabetes
*Observations*: Severe muscle tension and spasms extending through the entire back with pain, weak Spleen *qi*, Liver *qi* constraint, adrenal fatigue
*Illustrative treatment*: SP9, ST36, K3, LV3, LI4, LU7, LI11, CV12, BL10, BL40; Tight, tender points in the paraspinal muscles along both sides of the spine, levator scapula, trapezius

## Matt, Age 53
## Primary Complaint: Gout
## Secondary Complaints: Prostatitis, High Blood Pressure, High Cholesterol

Matt was a marketing executive and father of four children ages 12, 14, 18 and 20. Two of his kids were in college. He commuted four hours daily to and from work. On his train ride home each night he would have 2-3 drinks to unwind. On the weekends he ran intensely to burn off the stress.

When Matt came for acupuncture he was suffering from gouty arthritis in his left big toe joint. He also had prostatitis, causing intense burning pain in his lower abdomen. The gout made it difficult for him to put on his shoe and walk. He limped in to the office wearing only sandals and using a cane for support. He also suffered from both high blood pressure and high cholesterol and was taking medications to control them.

Matt's stress and exhausting schedule had caught up with him. Both of his pain conditions arose out of inflammation. His high blood pressure came from the same root cause – overwork, stress, and exhaustion. Treating it with medication was essential because sustained high blood pressure can lead to heart and kidney failure or stroke. However, other symptoms were bound to arise because the underlying condition was never treated.

He was highly stressed and fatigued, which was reflected in his pulses and body signs. His tongue was bright red, reflecting a lot of heat. His adrenal fatigue made him much less capable of fighting inflammation. His lifestyle was exhausting him more and more each day. Even his intense running regimen, which relaxed him, was too much exertion for his weak energetic condition, and was depleting him more.

Gout is much more common in men than in women. It is an inflammation of the joints, most often the big toe joint, associated with too much uric acid in the blood. This excess of uric acid may be related to excessive consumption of certain foods, including meat, as well as to high blood pressure, excessive alcohol intake, and excess fat and cholesterol in the blood.

I used points to restore balance in Matt's body, starting by strengthening the Kidneys, which includes the adrenals, the Spleen, Liver and Heart, and reducing inflammation. For the gout and prostatitis, in addition to acupuncture, I gave him an herbal formula to take at home, to help relieve the pain faster. I told about changing his diet, curtailing the alcohol consumption, and generally starting to think about how he could create a more balanced lifestyle and manage his stress in healthier ways. He wasn't able to run anyway due to the gout, but I asked him to consider another form of more gentle exercise while he was getting his strength back. Although he found it relaxing to run, it worked against his recovery by exhausting his already fatigued adrenals and entire body. He thought he could swim instead, and not push himself so hard, which was a good solution.

Because Matt was so highly motivated, realizing how dire his condition was, he arranged to take a full month off work to focus on his health. Fortunately, he was able to set this up with his employer. During that month we did two acupuncture treatments each week, Matt overhauled his diet, slept long hours at night without setting the alarm, took relaxing walks, read, swam and started meditating. He cut out alcohol altogether and changed his diet to more whole foods. Within a few days of his first treatment, the gout and prostatitis improved markedly, to the point of disappearing. By the end of the month Matt looked like a new person. Although he hadn't been very overweight, he had lost about 7 extra pounds without trying, he looked several years younger, and the redness was gone from his tongue along with the inflammation from his whole body. His blood pressure had gone down and he had consulted his doctor to reduce the medication levels. It seemed like he would soon be able to come off his medication altogether. All of his blood tests improved after the second month and his doctor allowed him to go off both the high blood pressure and cholesterol medications, because he didn't need them anymore.

When he returned to work, Matt consulted with his wife and together they agreed that he would reduce his weekly commute by staying at a hotel close to work a couple of nights a week. This allowed him time to rest and exercise, and when he took the train he used that time to work, enabling him to shorten his work hours in the office.

It is often a severe pain or disabling illness that serves as a wake up call for us to make changes. Matt said he wanted to get healthy and live to see his children grow, not to risk sudden or premature death from stress-induced disease. It is impressive to see how fast things can turn around by making the right changes. Matt's recovery was a great example of this.

*Symptoms*: Gouty arthritis pain in big toe, prostatitis, high blood pressure, high cholesterol
*Observations*: Red tongue, internal dampness and heat, inflammation, fatigue, weak Spleen, Kidneys, Heart, Liver
*Illustrative treatment*: LV4, LV8, K7, K10, ST36, SP9, LI11, PC4, Yintang, CV3, CV6, CV12, CV17

## Curtis, Age 62
## Primary Complaint: Enlarged Prostate with Frequent Urination
## Secondary Complaints: Knee Pain, Poor Sleep, Fatigue

Curtis came for acupuncture at his wife's suggestion to treat an enlarged prostate. His main problem was the prostate putting pressure on the bladder causing frequent urination, and his urinary flow was weak. Not only was that inconvenient during the day, but at night it woke him up almost every hour. He wasn't getting good sleep as a result and he was exhausted. He also suffered from pain and swelling in his right knee, which hurt when he walked, especially going up or down stairs. After examination and imaging, his doctor had attributed it to arthritis and prescribed anti-inflammatory medication.

Some degree of prostate enlargement is common to almost all men as they age. Curtis's pulses and body signs reflected weak Kidneys, corresponding in part to adrenal fatigue, and some damp heat, which is often found with conditions involving swellings or tissue enlargement and inflammation. Although Curtis's prostate was enlarged, he wasn't experiencing any symptoms of inflammation in the prostate but it was evident in his knee. Curtis's Spleen was also weak, contributing to his fatigue.

The way Curtis described it, he believed, as many people do, that his arthritis was a permanent diagnosis. In fact, arthritis simply means "joint inflammation" and it can have multiple causes, but in general it is the end result of pressure on a joint due to structural tension and strain, or injury.

In an arthritic joint there may also be joint degeneration, a wearing away of cartilage, or torn tendons or ligaments supporting the joint. Arthritis, left untreated, can lead to further joint degeneration. The joint inflammation can be relieved in most cases by resolving the muscle tension, strain or overuse that's causing it. This can be done using acupuncture and manual therapies. Acupuncture along with herbal and dietary remedies that relieve inflammation can also help in recovery from arthritis pain. If you're generating inflammation in your body through pro-inflammatory foods and stress, this conspires with the structural tension to produce greater joint inflammation.

I used acupuncture points to strengthen Curtis's underlying Kidney and Spleen weakness, and to clear dampness and heat. In addition to acupoints on the arms and legs, I used specific points surrounding the arthritic knee and others on the lower abdomen, followed by points on the lower back over the lower back and sacrum to move Blood and *qi* through the prostate area. I also treated the prostate point on the outer ear.

Curtis began to experience relief of his urinary frequency along with improved flow. Over the next four weeks he felt increasing energy and was only getting up once at night to urinate. His knee improved rapidly with reduced swelling and pain. After two months of acupuncture treatment, his knee felt completely normal most of the time. He occasionally aggravated it when climbing too many stairs in a day, but it quickly recovered each time.

> *Curtis began to experience relief of his urinary frequency along with improved flow. Over the next four weeks he felt increasing energy and was only getting up once at night to urinate. His knee improved rapidly with reduced swelling and pain.*

Acupuncture may not have eliminated Curtis's prostate enlargement, yet it reduced his symptoms to a minimal level and restored his quality of life. He continued to receive monthly acupuncture "maintenance" treatments to keep himself in good health and maintain the gains he had made in urinary and overall health.

*Symptoms*: Waking up frequently to urinate at night, fatigue, knee arthritis
*Observations*: Dampness and heat, inflammation of the knee, Spleen and Kidney *qi* deficiency, *qi* constraint, Blood stasis
*Illustrative treatment*: K7, LV5, "knee eyes," ST36, SP9, CV3, CV6, CV12, LI11, LI4, LU8, BL28, BL23, Outer sacrum, BL35, "prostate point" on ear

## Justin, Age 55
### Primary Complaint: Hemorrhoids
### Secondary Complaints: Constipation, Erectile Dysfunction

Justin worked long hours seated at his desk and in meetings and had painful hemorrhoids. He came to see if acupuncture could help him avoid surgery for the condition. Justin had suffered from long-term constipation. His internal signs pointed to weakness of the Spleen, with Large Intestine dryness, stasis of Blood and constrained Liver *qi*. Blood stasis means the blood doesn't move well enough and gets "stuck." This can contribute to dryness because the stuck Blood is unable to nourish and moisten the organs and tissues. Justin's constipation pattern was one of *qi* deficiency, dryness, *qi* constraint and Blood stasis.

I used acupuncture points to strengthen his Spleen and Kidneys, to get the Blood and *qi* moving, and to relieve dryness. I also used points known to help relieve constipation by activating the colon. I began with points on the arms and legs, and added points on the abdomen and later on the back, especially the lower back to treat the area of the colon and hemorrhoids. I advised Justin to get more movement, not only by exercising at the gym but by getting up and walking around more often at work. I also advised him on foods to help relieve constipation and gave him an herbal formula designed to move Blood, relieve hemorrhoids, and support smooth bowel movement. The doctor had advised him on soaking baths to relieve pain and swelling and had given him topical cream to apply, which he continued using.

Within a few days Justin had greatly relieved swelling and pain of hemorrhoids. He had two treatments the first week and then weekly treatments for another four weeks. After three weeks Justin mentioned that not only was the hemorrhoid pain gone and his constipation relieved, but his sexual function had greatly improved as well. He had struggled with erectile dysfunction for a few years but he didn't report it when he came for acupuncture –

> *After three weeks Justin mentioned that not only was the hemorrhoid pain gone and his constipation relieved, but his sexual function had greatly improved as well.*

in part because he didn't think it could help, and also because he was uncomfortable talking about it. When his virility improved markedly he knew it had to be the acupuncture. In fact, Justin's erectile dysfunction could be understood in terms of the same imbalances as his other problems – a lack of strength and flow of Blood and *qi*, especially in the pelvic region. By restoring healthy circulation of Blood and *qi* in this area, his erectile dysfunction resolved along with his other symptoms. Erectile dysfunction can arise from many different causes and in each case the patient is treated according to their individual patterns.

*Symptoms*: Painful hemorrhoids, erectile dysfunction
*Observations*: Weak Spleen and Kidneys, dryness in Large Intestine, *qi* constraint and Blood stasis
*Illustrative treatment*: GV20, GV4, BL35, BL25, BL23, BL20, BL18, BL17, BL13, home herbal medicine, dietary changes, exercise

## Keith, Age 42
## Primary Complaint: Snoring
## Secondary Complaints: Golfer's Elbow, Stress

Keith's snoring didn't bother him at all, but it kept his wife awake at night. He and his wife had two young children. Keith had a lot of stress, often working 10-12 hour days. He would have a couple of drinks at night to relax and then fall asleep hard, sleeping soundly through the night, but snoring loudly the entire time. He golfed almost every weekend unless there was snow on the ground and complained of "golfer's elbow" – tightness and pain near the right elbow – which he'd had for at least a year. His computer work seemed to aggravate it.

In Keith's pulses, tongue and body I found signs of Spleen and Kidney *qi* deficiency and Liver *qi* constraint. When there is snoring there is typically a weakness in the Spleen. Spleen deficiency is extremely common because it is exacerbated by overwork, overthinking, and irregular eating, including eating on the run. Because in acupuncture there is a relationship between the Spleen and the flesh or muscles, flaccidity in the tissue of the airways can be treated by strengthening the Spleen.

In Keith's case I also treated his Kidney *qi* and regulated the flow of energy through the Liver. These patterns help create the conditions that can lead to muscle and tendon strain. All of his imbalances traced back to his long work hours, high stress, eating irregularities and other lifestyle patterns including drinking alcohol to relax at night.

I used points on his arms, legs and abdomen, as well as points on the upper neck and head. For the golfer's elbow I treated acupoints directly on the tight muscles of the forearm and upper arm, and on the inflamed tendons around the elbow.

Keith noticed immediate relief of tension and pain in his elbow. I showed him stretches he could do to relax the muscles and avoid the strain that was causing tendonitis. I advised him to look at how he held the mouse and positioned his arm at the computer; even small movements can injure the tendon over time. By making changes in his computer posture and grip, he could take the stress off the arm. He needed four treatments on the elbow for complete relief of pain and tension in the area. Fortunately we did these treatments in the winter when he wasn't golfing, so the arm was getting some rest, and he made the recommended changes at the computer.

Keith's snoring gradually improved as we continued weekly treatments over the next six weeks. It was so much better that he rarely snored anymore at all, unless he'd had an exceptionally tiring week. If the snoring returned, he came back for an acupuncture treatment or two, until it went away again. While Keith's job and schedule remained demanding, he found ways to regulate the stress and to be more mindful of his need for rest and balance.

*Symptoms*: Snoring, "golfer's elbow" (tendonitis)
*Observations*: Weak Spleen and Kidney *qi*, Liver *qi* constraint with dampness and heat
*Illustrative treatment*: CV12, CV6, ST36, SP9, K3, LV3, LI4, LU7, GV20, Yintang, GB20; Trigger points: forearm extensors adjacent to elbow

## Kent, Age 30
## Primary Complaint: Insomnia
## Secondary Complaints: Stress, Insomnia, Anxiety

Kent was a young attorney with a very high pressure job. He was having difficulty sleeping because his mind was continuously chewing on his work and he stayed up late working. When he finally fell asleep, it was a light and disturbed sleep. He was waking up at 2 a.m. and was lucky if he could fall back to sleep, because his mind would start to race. He awakened frequently during the night and didn't feel rested in the morning.

Kent hoped that acupuncture could help with his anxiety and insomnia. He was soft-spoken and very polite. Smiling, he told me in a soft, restrained voice that the pressure builds up to the point where he feels like shouting. This was a very interesting way of expressing what he was feeling and pointed to his area of imbalance. The Liver is responsible for the smooth flow of energy in the body, and Liver *qi* is affected by stress, which obstructs its flow. Obstructed Liver *qi* generates anger, which comes out in the voice as a shout or a lack of shout—a kind of restrained flatness—and will tend to waken you at around 2 a.m.

Palpating his pulses, abdomen, and meridians and looking at his tongue all confirmed the pattern of constrained Liver *qi*. There was also a deficiency of Spleen *qi*, most likely exacerbated by the Liver imbalance. Spleen deficiency both arises from and causes over-thinking, worry, and pensiveness. The Kidneys were deficient as well, corresponding in part to Kent's relentless adrenal stress, and there was excess *qi* trapped in the Heart. All of these patterns must be treated together, and I selected the points on this basis.

I suggested to Kent that he learn to meditate. I spoke about the value of harnessing the power of his mind and not letting it run his life. The stress of his job was unlikely to change; he needed to learn skills for managing it more effectively. In a subsequent session I showed him how to do a simple meditation with the breath, which he could do for a few minutes a day.

I find that people at around age 30 are ready to refine their way of living and cultivate greater mastery of life skills. Until this time, they've been starting their careers and trying their best to prove their worth while learning the ropes. At 30 they have begun to realize that while they can survive by pushing their bodies hard to achieve a goal, now it's time to go beyond plain survival and develop skills for greater mastery and enjoyment of life. Usually, as in Kent's case, their bodies have broken down in one way or another, through fatigue, pain syndromes, anxiety, and insomnia, and they find they cannot continue in the way they've been going. It's time for a change.

In addition to acupuncture and meditation, I suggested other ways for Kent to support his mind to stop its excessive brooding and worrying. Starting with what and how he ate, Kent could begin to strengthen his Spleen. I suggested two simple actions to start with: first, sit down and eat meals without working or meeting or facing the computer screen; second, chew and breathe while eating. Third, I suggested not letting too much time pass between meals. He confessed that he could go for an entire day without eating because of his frantic schedule. He also didn't drink water for much of the day. It really wouldn't take much to adjust these habits and in doing so he would be healing his own body and helping to calm his own mind.

Kent needed regular exercise to help move the blocked Liver *qi*. He was getting to the gym mainly on weekends. We talked about what he could do each day to move energy in his body. By moving his body and using his breath, he would be doing another "self-treatment" and moving that blocked *qi*, thereby releasing the stress pattern. He suggested that he could do twenty minutes of exercise at home before leaving for work, and he could also walk to work more frequently, weather permitting, instead of taking the train. So he came up with some effective strategies for treating his own imbalances and resolving his insomnia and stress, within the structure of a very demanding job.

*Symptoms*: Anxiety, insomnia, waking nightly at 2 a.m., fatigue
*Observations*: Dry, red tongue with redder tip and edges, constrained *qi* of Liver and Heart, weak Spleen
*Illustrative treatment*: K4, PC4, LV3, SP9, ST36, LI11, CV17, Yintang

## John, Age 68
## Primary Complaint: Lower Back Pain, Sciatica, Stenosis
## Secondary Complaint: Shoulder Pain

John was a very active and fit business executive. However, he was having lower back pain and shooting pain down his right leg. His doctor had ordered an MRI of the lower back, which revealed some disc degeneration and stenosis in the lumbar spine. This compressed the nerves coming from the lower back down the leg, causing leg pain and tingling. His doctor didn't think it was severe enough to warrant surgery and prescribed physical therapy instead, which hadn't helped much. In spite of the doctor's reassurance, the MRI report, written in medical jargon, sounded ominous. John was very concerned about his condition. He worried that it would only worsen over time and curtail his exercise—biking, skiing, and working out at the gym.

My initial exam showed that John was internally strong and well-balanced for his age. There was some depletion in the Kidney and Spleen, involving the adrenals and the digestion. Weakened Kidneys correspond to problems with the bones and lower back. His lower back muscles were extremely tight, as were his gluteal and piriformis muscles, which support the pelvis and hip. Although the pain was on his left side, John noted that the pain had started in the right hip and then changed sides. This makes more sense than it may appear; the two sides of the pelvis and hips are meant to be level, and if one side is pulled "out" the other side is bound to respond by going out as well. Frequently the symptomatic side is not where the problem started. The body's structural relationships have to be evaluated to find the source of the problem to treat it effectively. If you only treat the symptom but not the source, your results will be limited.

I chose points to strengthen John's Spleen and Kidney *qi*, while directly relieving muscle tension using trigger point release in the lower back, hips, and legs, wherever I found it through palpation. John followed a series of home exercises to help balance, stretch, and strengthen his back and legs. He was quickly relieved of the leg pain and began to learn how to balance his own body. The pain started to clear up. He discovered that if he began to feel the leg tingling during the day, all he had to do was stretch out his lower back and it would stop immediately. He returned to biking and all his normal exercise and no longer feared that his condition would worsen and inhibit him. Gaining both an intellectual and physical understanding of his imbalance and how to treat it was an essential component in John's healing, one that allowed him to play an active role in remaining pain-free and staying fit.

*Symptoms*: Lower back pain, shooting pain and tingling down the leg
*Observations*: Disc compression, spinal stenosis, structural imbalance with tension in the lower back, hips, legs, and shoulder, internal weakness in the Kidneys and Spleen
*Illustrative treatment*: BL40, BL10, BL60, BL58, BL23, BL20, K7, Vertebral points at L1 through L5, Trigger points: quadratus lumborum, lumbar paraspinals, gluteus medius, piriformis

# CHAPTER FOUR

...................

# Acupuncture: An Ancient Healing Technique

"Study the past if you would define the future."
—Confucius

It's hard to imagine how the idea first occurred to someone: "Hey, let's stick a needle in that and see if it heals the patient." No one really knows who first thought of it and why. We may never know for certain how the use of needles to treat acupuncture points first began.

However, we can piece together a plausible hypothesis based on archeological evidence and existing acupuncture manuscripts, principally the *Neijing*.[1] Also known as *The Yellow Emperor's Classic of Chinese Medicine*, the *Neijing* dates to the 2nd century BCE. It is attributed to Huang Di, the legendary Yellow Emperor of ancient China, and is the oldest known manuscript on the principles and practice of acupuncture.

The Yellow Emperor is said to have reigned around the third millennium BCE, more than 2,500 years ago. A mythical figure to whom many great innovations and accomplishments in Chinese history are ascribed, it's unknown whether the Huang Di was an actual historical figure or not. If he did exist, he probably didn't write the *Neijing*.[2] Because older ideas were given greater credence in ancient China than newer ones, the *Neijing* is believed to be a compendium of medical knowledge that was added to over the course of many centuries, attributed to the Yellow Emperor, and then restored and edited in the 8th century CE.[3]

The *Neijing* takes the form of a dialogue between Huang Di and his ministers. Because it is a compilation of ideas that was added to over the centuries, it contains multiple explanations that often conflict or contradict one another and at other times overlap and agree.[4]

## Acupuncture in China: Past and Present

The system of thought and medicine that gave rise to acupuncture may go back as far as 5,000 years. Yet, the earliest evidence of needles being used for therapeutic treatment of acupuncture points dates only to the second century BCE. In addition to written texts discussing acupuncture dating to that time, ancient artifacts – gold and silver acupuncture needles – were unearthed in 1968 in a Chinese tomb dating to 113 BCE.[5]

We simply don't know how far back needles were used for acupuncture treatment, or how they might have developed out of earlier tools – sharpened stones and bones – that were used for lancing and bloodletting, possibly even to chase out "demons" in shamanic healing. Before the use of needles, acupuncture points were treated with heat by burning herbs over the skin – usually mugwort – a practice known as "moxibustion" which is still used today.

> *The system of thought and medicine that gave rise to acupuncture may go back as far as 5,000 years. Yet, the earliest evidence of needles being used for therapeutic treatment of acupuncture points dates only to the second century BCE.*

Over time, acupuncturists devised various needling techniques to enhance their effects: using needles made of different metals – including gold, silver, copper, and bronze; heating the needles; inserting them in the direction of or against the meridian flow; inserting or removing needles when the patient inhales or exhales, and so on.

Ancient acupuncturists observed that changes in the feel, appearance or sensitivity in specific locations on the body's surface could be found when a particular organ was diseased. When selected points were needled using acupuncture, a characteristic sensation of soreness or electricity would be propagated along distinct pathways and felt by the patient. Even today these pathways can be felt and described in a replicable way by patients receiving acupuncture. The treatment of acupuncture points was observed to affect not only diseased organs, but also other parts of the body far from the point or the organ.

By making observations like these, the ancient acupuncturists were able to develop knowledge of the therapeutic effects of specific acupuncture points and the system of meridians that connected them.

Acupuncture's popularity in China has fluctuated over the centuries, going in and out of favor with the ruling and upper classes. During the Song Dynasty (960-1279 CE), it is said that Emperor Renzong was successfully cured of an ailment through the use of acupuncture. It was during this period that life-size bronze statues depicting the points were created as a teaching tool, and acupuncture was accorded greater respect as a medical treatment.

By the 17th century acupuncture had again fallen out of favor, giving way to an emphasis on tuina massage and herbal medicine as preferred methods of treatment, particularly among the upper classes. Acupuncture was even banned by China's rulers from the curriculum of medical colleges for a time, although it was still passed down through family lineages and remained in use by common people.

Not until the latter half of the 20th century did acupuncture enjoy a revival in China, and this happened only by chance you might say. Communist Party leaders had strongly rejected traditional Chinese medicine, including acupuncture, as being backward and superstitious, and favored the use of Western-style scientific medicine. But with limited access to modern medical tools, having no other options, Mao Tse Tung reversed this position. Under his direction, acupuncture and herbal medicine enjoyed a resurgence. "Barefoot Doctors" were trained in acupuncture and dispatched to villages throughout China to provide acute medical care to the rural populace. The ancient practice of Chinese medicine was revived and put to use for practical purposes.

As acupuncture came back into use, a significant change took place in the way it was practiced. Its underlying philosophy was revised to reflect the more materialistic values of the Marxist ruling party. The broad range of practice styles that had developed over thousands of years was distilled into one officially sanctioned version of acupuncture. What emerged is what is known today as "Traditional Chinese Medicine" or TCM. It is the version of acupuncture that was developed in the 1950s and 1960s under Chairman Mao.

It would be natural to assume that acupuncture as presently taught and practiced in China represents the "purest" form of acupuncture, but this is not the case. TCM, like other styles of acupuncture that developed in other countries over time, is a variant version of acupuncture, influenced by the culture, philosophy, and beliefs of the time and place.

The official use of acupuncture in China today tends to be highly medicalized. Here in the U.S. we view it more as an alternative "non-medical" approach, aimed at restoring health from the inside out in the context of "wellness." Consequently, Western acupuncture today is not identical to contemporary acupuncture in China, and both differ from ancient Chinese acupuncture as practiced centuries ago.

Acupuncture has always adapted to the place and time in which it is used. Different styles of acupuncture are associated with Japan, Korea, Vietnam, and different regions of China. In line with this tradition, Western acupuncture is cultivated in the field of our own outlook and needs.[6]

While its core principles are shared among all styles, each variant maintains its own characteristics, much like dialects of the same language that evolve and diverge in unique ways. China is best known for

> *Acupuncture has always adapted to the place and time in which it is used. Different styles of acupuncture are associated with Japan, Korea, Vietnam, and different regions of China. In line with this tradition, Western acupuncture is cultivated in the field of our own outlook and needs.*

the system of acupuncture and widely considered to be its point of origin; however, there is some fascinating evidence suggesting that acupuncture may also have been used in ancient Egypt, India, and Persia.[7] One can only speculate about how such knowledge may have been carried by migration across trade routes in pre-recorded history.

# Acupuncture: Prevention or Cure?

From the beginning, acupuncture's philosophical emphasis was on early treatment to prevent rather than cure illness. Yet, in practice, acupuncture was used to treat a wide range of illnesses. Because it promotes the body's own self-healing abilities, it can serve both purposes.

Traditional herbal medicine was, and still is, used alongside acupuncture. In contrast to acupuncture, in which prevention was emphasized, Chinese herbal medicine was oriented towards relieving symptoms and prolonging life, with an ideal of possibly achieving immortality. Herbal medicine, while it has distinct differences from pharmaceutical medicine as we know it today, is somewhat related to it. While acupuncture uses only needles, heat and pressure, herbal medicine uses bioactive chemical substances taken internally to heal illness and restore health.

Other approaches to healing that were traditionally used in conjunction with acupuncture include massage and joint manipulation (tuina), moxibustion (treating acupoints with heat), cupping (using suction cups to promote circulation), gua sha (stroking the skin with a firm object), bone setting, breathing exercises (qigong), physical exercise and stretching, as well as dietary therapy. Most of these, apart from extensive joint manipulation and bone setting, are within the scope of present day acupuncture practice in the U.S.

# Acupuncture in the West

Acupuncture initially made its way to Europe in the 17th century, brought by missionaries returning from China. In the United States, small numbers of Chinese immigrants are known to have practiced it as early as the nineteenth century. But its first major exposure was in 1971 when James Reston, a journalist for the *New York Times*, reported his own experience of receiving acupuncture for post-operative pain after undergoing an emergency appendectomy in Beijing.[8]

Shortly thereafter, in 1972, President Richard Nixon visited China, and acupuncture was again featured in American news reports. Subsequently, interest in acupuncture began to grow in the United States and in the years that followed it became legalized and licensed as a profession throughout the country.

Over the past forty years or so, an increasing number of scientific studies have been conducted on the efficacy and mechanisms of acupuncture treatment. In 1997, the National Institutes of Health (NIH) issued a consensus statement on acupuncture that concluded, "There is sufficient evidence of acupuncture's value to expand its use into conventional medicine and to encourage further studies of its physiology and clinical value."[9] Accordingly, NIH provides funding for U.S.-based studies into the mechanisms and effectiveness of acupuncture. Similar studies are also being carried out in China and other parts of the world.

> *In 1997, the National Institutes of Health (NIH) issued a consensus statement on acupuncture that concluded, "There is sufficient evidence of acupuncture's value to expand its use into conventional medicine and to encourage further studies of its physiology and clinical value."*

In 2003, several years after the NIH consensus statement, the World Health Organization (WHO) listed forty-three diseases, symptoms, and conditions for which acupuncture had proven effective, based on a review of controlled clinical studies. It further listed sixty-three diseases and conditions that had been shown to respond to acupuncture but for which further proof was needed.[10] I have treated nearly all of these conditions in my own acupuncture practice over the years with good results and I am confident that I could treat most of them successfully.

In contemporary China, acupuncture and herbal medicine are practiced not only in privately run clinics but also in hospitals.[11] A small but growing number of hospitals in the United States now provide acupuncture and herbal medicine to patients as well.[12] Most commonly in the U.S., acupuncture is found in private clinics run by one or a small group of acupuncturists working together. It is also available in acupuncture student clinics and in community clinics that offer non-private acupuncture treatments in group settings for reduced rates. Acupuncture is increasingly found within integrative medical clinics that combine conventional and alternative medicine and in medical fertility practices. It is also used for narrower applications in drug addiction treatment facilities to help patients withdraw from substance abuse and increasingly for veterans suffering from post-traumatic stress disorder.

Acupuncture's many forms of expression may be considered part of its strength as a medicine. Globalization, and the resulting exchange of knowledge, has enabled the best of the acupuncture traditions to come together. At the same time, acupuncture is coming into direct contact with Western science and medicine, stimulating yet another level of creative inquiry, investigation and dialogue.

## Acupuncture Anesthesia?

Media reports going back to the 1970s have sensationalized the notion of acupuncture being used for anesthesia during surgery in place of drugs. The use of acupuncture alone for the purpose of anesthesia is not considered to be an effective substitute for conventional anesthesia.[13] It was evidently attempted in China, possibly for political reasons, to show the West the superiority of Chinese medicine, or for financial reasons, to try to provide surgery to large numbers of people who could not afford conventional anesthesia. There may have been some deceptive demonstrations showing acupuncture being used for anesthesia in Chinese surgeries while standard medical anesthesia was surreptitiously administered during the procedure.

> *Media reports going back to the 1970s have sensationalized the notion of acupuncture being used for anesthesia during surgery in place of drugs. The use of acupuncture alone for the purpose of anesthesia is not considered to be an effective substitute for conventional anesthesia.*

In China, the combined use of acupuncture and drugs in surgery is to this day being researched as a way to control costs. Some research suggests that this approach may be viable and that it can possibly minimize post-operative side effects from the more powerful general anesthesia drugs.[14]

However, acupuncture anesthesia is not in use for surgical procedures in the United States. Interestingly, among the many American health insurance providers that cover acupuncture, I have come across a few that allow it "only when used for anesthesia." I can only surmise that this is a way to deceive subscribers into thinking they have acupuncture coverage when they do not. Either that or the policy was written without any thought or study of the subject. Most insurance plans that cover acupuncture do so for real medical conditions, primarily pain.

## Key Points

- Acupuncture's system of thought may have originated 5,000 years ago or earlier.
- The earliest evidence of acupuncture needles being used for treatment dates to about 2,200 years ago.
- Moxibustion was used to treat acupoints before the development of acupuncture needles.
- Before the use of needles, therapeutic treatment was performed using sharpened stones and bones. It is not known whether these tools were used on acupuncture points or mainly to pierce boils and abscesses and for bloodletting.
- The Neijing, from the 2nd century BCE, is the oldest known acupuncture manuscript.
- Acupuncture has gone in and out of favor in China over the course of its history.
- Mao Tse Tung revived the practice of acupuncture in the mid-20th century.
- Modern day acupuncture in China is a recently developed style known as TCM ("Traditional Chinese Medicine").
- Acupuncture was originally conceived as a preventive wellness treatment but was also used for treatment of illness.
- Herbal medicine was used alongside acupuncture with a greater emphasis on relieving symptoms and prolonging life.

- Acupuncture is one element of the complete system of Chinese medicine which also includes herbal medicine, tuina massage, moxibustion, cupping, gua sha, bone setting, qi gong breathing exercises, physical exercise, and dietary therapy.
- Acupuncture was made popular in the United States in the early 1970s.
- The National Institutes of Health (NIH) supports the scientific study of acupuncture.
- The World Health Organization (WHO) has endorsed acupuncture for the treatment of over 63 conditions.
- Acupuncture is not used in place of anesthesia for surgery.
- Acupuncture is practiced in private clinics, community clinics, acupuncture college clinics, integrative medical clinics, in some hospitals and in centers for treatment of addictions as well as for veterans.

CHAPTER FIVE

· · · · · · · · · · · · · · · · · · · · ·

# The Science of Acupuncture

"Nothing in life is to be feared, it is only to be understood. Now
is the time to understand more, so that we may fear less."
—Marie Curie

It is perhaps a measure of how disconnected we feel that we are so skeptical
and turn to science to prove what, in a sense, is self-evident. By design, the
human body is elegantly interconnected. Each one of us started out as a
single cell that grew into a fully differentiated person who lives, breathes,
eats, gets sick, gets well again, and eventually dies. The entire "program"
for our growth, development, healing and eventual decline and death exists
within that one single cell. Why, then, are we so incredulous that every part
of us interconnects with every other part, that a cell in our toe might have
a way of relating to one in our arm or in our brain? At what point do we
assume that the intelligence of that one initial cell broke down and caused
our bodies to stop being so brilliant and interconnected?

Acupuncture recognizes the body's integrity: every part "communicates"
and connects with every other part. Beyond that, acupuncture theory
considers human experience as more than physical: we have emotions,
thoughts, and spirit, and these lie on a continuum with the physical body.
Just as water has phases including solid (ice), liquid and vapor, human
beings have physical, emotional, mental and spiritual phases that are all
part of one greater whole.

Western science is beginning to reveal evidence that supports the
hypothesis of interconnectivity of the body, mind, and emotions. We take

for granted that we salivate at the thought of delicious food when we're hungry. That's a physical reaction produced by a thought or the aroma of food. Similarly, when we're nervous before a test, an interview, or a performance, it's common for us to react with a racing heart and sweaty palms. The body's ability to translate stress into hormonal signals, neurochemical modulation, changes in mood and energy, and even changes in genetic expression, is beyond dispute. It is also proven that a stimulus to any part of the body can produce measurable changes in the brain. We live this experience every day in so many ways. Why is it so difficult for us to imagine that an acupuncture needle placed in the hand might relieve head pain, toothache, acid reflux or even tendonitis?

The concept of spirit is even more of a reach in science and therefore relegated to the realm of religion most of the time; yet science has shown that deep states of meditation and the transcendent experience of spiritual ecstasy can be measured in the brain and body. Researchers at Harvard University have demonstrated that meditation reduces the occurrence of specific changes in our DNA that are correlated with aging. Meditators also produced much lower levels of disease-causing inflammatory chemicals in their bodies. These changes were found even in beginning meditators after only eight weeks.[1]

Many indigenous cultures depend on an awareness of human existence as part of a greater whole. Native American tradition is replete with stories reflecting this: spirits of nature and animals were invoked in ritual with reverence and respect. They used herbs as medicine to treat ailments and disease. Now we tend to look askance at herbal remedies as "untested" or "unproven." Lab tests and clinical trials are done to validate their efficacy, and isolated ingredients are prepared as "standardized extracts" to receive the scientific stamp of approval. In so doing we may

> *Researchers at Harvard University have demonstrated that meditation reduces the occurrence of specific changes in our DNA that are correlated with aging. Meditators also produced much lower levels of disease-causing inflammatory chemicals in their bodies. These changes were found even in beginning meditators after only eight weeks.*

be removing hundreds of other active ingredients within an herb, but we trust what is known through science and distrust all else. Maybe this gives us a sense of control and security in an uncontrollable, incomprehensible universe, but we may be inadvertently losing something valuable in the process.

We are enmeshed in a larger web of existence: seasons, the weather, sunlight and darkness affect us differently, depending on our internal constitution. We are interconnected with our environment. Science may not yet have evidence to explain all of it, but we know it from our own experience. In acupuncture it's understood that a person with a "damp" condition will suffer more in humid conditions; a person who is internally "cold" will not do well in winter; and a person suffering from conditions of "wind," including itching and sneezing and twitches, will feel worse in spring, the season associated with wind in acupuncture. These correspondences don't seem so strange once we apply our own experience.

## Can Science Explain Acupuncture?

In reviewing the status of acupuncture research to date, I must admit to loving the science. I enjoy the process by which experiments are designed and carried out. It's thrilling to discover – through experimentation – the body's elegant, complex, and highly intelligent functions.

Scientific validation can help to make acupuncture more widely available, while reducing health care costs both individually and collectively, and it may help to refine or innovate new treatments for certain diseases. Nevertheless, science may never provide us with a fully satisfying explanation of how acupuncture really works. Why? Because science is linear, while the body's integrated functions – and the concepts of acupuncture – are nonlinear.

*Scientific validation can help to make acupuncture more widely available, while reducing health care costs both individually and collectively, and it may help to refine or innovate new treatments for certain diseases.*

Countless simultaneous processes are occurring in our bodies every millisecond. Each "input" into our system—whether it's cold or heat, hunger or thirst, frustration, grief, infection, fatigue, anger, joy, pain, injury, rest, aging or any number of infinite variables—induces whole-system responses that are far-reaching and complex. Some are measurable with our tools and knowledge, and others are not. Science is always finding new, smaller particles and properties of energy that were previously unknown. The human body is functioning in ways as yet beyond our understanding. We are limited by the questions we ask, the kinds of experiments we design, and by our instruments, including our own minds.

In this chapter, I want to examine the science of acupuncture, because it is so fascinating as well as validating. I'm very grateful to those scientists whose dedicated efforts are providing us with valuable research data. And yet, reviewing the science has reaffirmed my personal decision to practice acupuncture clinically rather than wait for the results of scientific research. I see patients every day struggling to find balance in their lives, an experience of wholeness and healing that goes beyond taking a pill. Scientific explanations alone do not make people feel better or heal more quickly. More people want to restore a sense of integration to their lives and their health, and for this, many are turning to acupuncture. And while it is not the answer to everything, acupuncture remains an accessible, potent, and virtually harmless technique that can heal and restore the balance that people are seeking, not after months or years but in days and weeks.

I think you'll find some of what I've learned about the current science of acupuncture compelling. It won't provide all the answers yet. In reviewing scientifically proven effects of acupuncture, it is essential to recognize that all of the observed effects – in the nervous system, brain, hormones and so on – while providing evidence of what is happening, do not tell us *how* acupuncture really works. We are moving towards an understanding of acupuncture's effects and possible mechanisms, and we can postulate theories, but we can't yet say conclusively how it works, or prove beyond a doubt its effectiveness for all conditions.

# Acupuncture Scientific Research

There are different approaches to scientific research.

- *Basic research* takes scientific measurements using experimental human or animal subjects in the lab.
- *Randomized controlled trials* are studies using humans – either healthy volunteers or patients suffering from a specific disorder – to measure clinical treatment effects.
- A third approach uses *systematic reviews*, in which researchers use data from multiple studies to make broad statements about acupuncture's effectiveness.

In acupuncture trials to date, the research design is often lacking, and the studies aren't standardized in a way that would support comparison of results. In large part, this is due to an insufficient ability to control for variables (since we don't know all the variables). In addition, we're not sure how well research trials compare with clinical practice.

Sham acupuncture – needling non-acupuncture points – is frequently used as a control to test the effects of true acupuncture points. Since we don't yet know how acupuncture needles cause their effects, we can't be sure that non-acupuncture points will be neutral; in fact, research suggests that they are not.[2] Also, scientific trials aim to eliminate elements of the clinical acupuncture encounter, such as palpation of pulse or meridians, which may themselves have therapeutic influences.[3]

Sometimes these shortcomings are overcome, at least in part, by combining results from multiple research studies in a systematic review. This method has the ability to reveal trends over a wide range of studies. Its weakness is that it depends on the quality of the original studies to a great extent and is subject to bias. A specific type of systematic review is known as a *meta-analysis*. In this approach, statistical tools are used to evaluate pooled results from multiple studies, and this can minimize the influence of poorly designed studies.

In a recent meta-analysis studying acupuncture for osteoarthritis of the knee, for example, researchers determined that acupuncture was significantly better at relieving pain and restoring function than sham acupuncture, standard care treatment, or no treatment at all.[4] For most conditions we don't yet have the benefit of a meta-analysis proving acupuncture's efficacy. Instead, we are working from individual studies that demonstrate acupuncture's effects.

In going through the literature, one can choose to cherry-pick those research studies that demonstrate a proven effect or those that seem to disprove it. One can try to be unbiased and display all of them and then conclude that "more research is needed"—which is what most reviews say in the end.

What I'm going to do is present what I find most interesting and useful in understanding acupuncture. I've selected research studies on a few illustrative conditions which, while perhaps not yet providing a comprehensive explanation, are well-designed and provide substantial proof of acupuncture's effects. This is acupuncture science viewed through the lens of a biochemist-turned-acupuncturist.

> *In a recent meta-analysis studying acupuncture for osteoarthritis of the knee, for example, researchers determined that acupuncture was significantly better at relieving pain and restoring function than sham acupuncture, standard care treatment, or no treatment at all.*

## Acupuncture's Natural High

When people come for acupuncture, especially for the first time, I advise them about what to expect immediately after treatment: "You're going to feel spaced out, like you're on a natural high. Watch your step as you walk, hold the handrails on the stairs, and move more slowly than usual."

We've had some comical experiences in the reception area as patients prepare to leave after a visit. Some try to pay with their metro fare card; others can't seem to collect their belongings to walk out the door while smiling and laughing. Once, two women ended up with each other's coats (they met up to exchange them later!). There's a lot of laughter and giddiness. As it turns out, science can help to explain this.

Acupuncture induces the release of endorphins, our body's natural painkillers. Also known as opioids, they are chemically related to substances derived from the poppy plant, such as opium and morphine. In addition to relieving pain, these opioids induce feelings of euphoria. When acupuncture patients come out of treatment feeling euphoric as if on a "natural high," this is quite literally true. Unlike artificial "highs," induced by harmful drugs, the natural high induced by acupuncture is actually our innate state of balance and wellness.

## Using Acupuncture to Treat Pain

Pain is the most obvious condition to study. Several decades ago, researchers used cerebrospinal fluid from rabbits they'd treated with acupressure, and injected it into untreated rabbits, where it produced analgesic effects.[5] This indicated that a biochemical agent was involved – induced by acupressure – which could be transferred from one rabbit to another through fluid.

Subsequent research has involved both laboratory experiments and clinical trials that attempt to quantify pain relief in actual patients.[6] The research data become detailed very quickly. For example, depending on the way the acupuncture needle is stimulated once inserted – manually, or with low or high frequency electro-stimulation, different types of opioids are released.[7] This is consistent with traditional acupuncture's assertion that there are various methods of needle manipulation, each with its own effects, which must be selected appropriately for each patient and each individual acupoint.

When acupuncture signals reach the brain, multiple regions in the brain are activated and some are deactivated.[8] Different acupoints are shown to affect different areas in the brain, even when those acupoints are located in the region of the same spinal segment.[9]

Because the body's functions are both elegantly orchestrated and complex, there are at least two different pathways mediating acupuncture's pain-relieving effects: one is neural (involving the nervous system), and the other is hormonal.[10]

The neural pathway is the one in which signals are sent via the nerves to the spinal cord and brain, causing the release of natural painkilling substances.

The hormonal pathway has a different effect: it relieves inflammation. It works via a set of endocrine glands known as the hypothalamus-pituitary-adrenal (HPA) axis. These three glands work together in complex ways to regulate multiple body functions, one of which is anti-inflammatory. Acupuncture causes a "hormone cascade," ultimately releasing corticosterone— one of the body's natural anti-inflammatory substances—from the adrenal glands.[11]

> *Because the body's functions are both elegantly orchestrated and complex, there are at least two different pathways mediating acupuncture's pain-relieving effects: one is neural (involving the nervous system), and the other is hormonal.*

This much we know: acupuncture stimulates the body's release of natural painkillers through the spinal cord and brain. At the same time, it generates the release of natural anti-inflammatory substances through the hormonal system. A third set of cellular chemical reactions happens at the site of needling, involving release of locally-mediated tissue healing and pain-relieving substances as well as connective tissue responses.[12] These scientific data provide evidence of at least some of the specific pathways through which acupuncture treats both pain and inflammation.

## Lower Back Pain

In a study of patients with spinal stenosis and lumbar disc herniation causing lower back and sciatic pain down the leg, acupuncture was tested in five locations:

1. Adjacent to the affected disc;
2. At the pudendal nerve (located in the pelvis);
3. At the sciatic nerve (which runs from the lower back through the pelvis into the leg);

4. In the lumbar muscles;
5. At the nerve root, which emerges from the spinal cord.

Researchers assessed improvement on the basis of the following:

• Reduced pain;
• Increased continuous walking distance;
• Increased blood flow.

Each of the points was found effective to varying degrees. About half of the patients were effectively relieved of pain using the acupoint adjacent to the problem disc. Electro-acupuncture on the pudendal nerve relieved the symptoms that hadn't responded to the disc-adjacent point. Significant, sustained pain relief was also found after electro-acupuncture was applied at the nerve root.

In an animal study using rats, sciatic nerve blood flow was increased by over 50 percent in response to acupuncture at the lumbar muscles, and by 100 percent when administered to the pudendal nerve or the sciatic nerve.[13] This research suggests that acupuncture may help by improving blood flow to the nerve root and sciatic nerve, in addition to inhibiting pain via the nervous system.

The proof of results in rats – and not only humans – rules out the placebo effect as potentially being the sole cause, as the rats can have no expectation for acupuncture's ability to change their physiology.

## Carpal Tunnel Syndrome

This syndrome is a common pain condition affecting the wrist and hand. The median nerve becomes entrapped as it passes through the wrist due to pressure from surrounding soft tissue, causing paresthesia (tingling or other abnormal sensations) and pain in the first four fingers.

Researchers used functional magnetic resonance imaging (fMRI) of the brain in carpal tunnel patients and found that the brain regions representing the affected fingers were altered.

These patients displayed hyperactivation of the brain in response to mild sensory stimulation of the affected fingers, and expanded representation of these fingers in the brain. There was also blurring of the brain regions corresponding to two adjacent fingers.

After five weeks of acupuncture treatments to the affected wrist and arm in carpal tunnel patients, the brain representations of the fingers returned to normal positions and were no longer blurred or hyperactivated by stimulation to the fingers. These brain changes correlated with the patients' reduced paresthesia and pain.[14]

These findings are especially significant since conventional treatments for carpal tunnel syndrome – involving wrist splints or surgery – are either ineffective or highly invasive and expensive. Surgery is the definitive treatment and results in pain relief as great as 90 percent. However, follow-up studies suggest that surgery patients fare no better in the long term than those treated more conservatively.

Acupuncture for carpal tunnel syndrome is cost-effective, minimally invasive, potentially longer lasting, and easily repeatable if needed.

## Neuropathic Pain

Acupuncture has been studied for the treatment of neuropathic pain, which is poorly understood even in Western medicine. This kind of pain arises from various conditions—surgery, disease, or as a side effect of chemotherapy or certain medications—and may result in numbness or unusual sensations, known as allodynia.

In one study, two acupuncture points were tested for their ability to relieve allodynia in rats. The findings showed that both points significantly relieved allodynia, but that each acupoint relieved different aspects of the pain. The type of pain induced by touch was reduced by needling acupoint ST-36, located on the outer leg, while another type of pain, induced by cold, was reduced by

*Many studies on acupuncture pain relief reveal that multiple mechanisms of analgesia, or pain relief, are involved, including both local and central nervous system effects. The type of stimulation applied to the acupuncture point determines which of these mechanisms is activated.*

needling acupoint SP-9, located on the inner leg, and each case the pain relief was statistically significant when compared to the control groups.[15]

Many studies on acupuncture pain relief reveal that multiple mechanisms of analgesia, or pain relief, are involved, including both local and central nervous system effects. The type of stimulation applied to the acupuncture point influences which of these mechanisms is activated.

In this study, both points were manually stimulated in precisely the same manner, suggesting that the points have different specific effects. This indicates that point selection in an acupuncture treatment also influences which mechanisms of pain relief are activated. In acupuncture theory this is a given; individual points have specific functions.

## Beyond Pain Relief: Using Acupuncture to Treat Other Disorders

In addition to the opioids, nerve fibers, and brain regions involved, scientists have identified quite a few other naturally-occurring chemicals in the body that are stimulated by acupuncture.[16] Each of these substances interacts with unique receptor molecules on the surface of cells to trigger biochemical reactions that mediate pain and other conditions. These include non-opioid neurotransmitters such as serotonin and gamma-aminobutyric acid (GABA) – both of which have known functions in the brain and body, including mood and energy regulation. In fact, serotonin is known to be involved in the regulation of depression. Since we know that acupuncture can measurably affect serotonin in the brain and body, we can begin to imagine one way it might work in relieving depression.

### Depression

Depression is a complex condition that may arise from multiple causes.[17] Some patients may suffer from a genetic predisposition to it. With or without this tendency, patients can become depressed due to life events, illness, injury, pregnancy or postpartum changes. The etiology of depression as a symptom is not well understood. The most widely used anti-depressant medications are selective serotonin reuptake inhibitors

(SSRIs), based on the clinical observation that more available serotonin in the brain is correlated with reduced depression.[18]

Anti-depressants are among the most highly prescribed medications in the U.S. In conventional medical care, anti-depressants are often combined with psychotherapy to treat clinical depression, which is associated with a chemical imbalance in the brain but is frequently connected to emotional and psychological factors in a patient's life.

People often turn to acupuncture to help alleviate depression. Clinical studies provide evidence in support of acupuncture's efficacy in treating it. In my own experience with depressed patients seeking help through acupuncture, I have seen good results in most cases. But there's a caveat: the depressed patients who respond best to acupuncture are the ones who engage in multiple approaches to treatment, using psychotherapy, nutrition, herbal medicine, exercise, meditation, and appropriate lifestyle changes. Many patients arrive for their first acupuncture treatment already using a prescription antidepressant. After a period of acupuncture treatments, they often find that they are able to wean off the medication with their doctor's support.

Critics might argue that this does nothing to support the claim that acupuncture relieves depression. They could say that lifestyle changes, along with the placebo effect, are what alleviate the symptoms. Most of the clinical trials for acupuncture treatment of depression in humans are too variable to be of use in drawing firm conclusions. In animal models evidence has shown distinct anti-depressant effects, but it is unknown how comparable the stress-induced depression in lab rats is to different forms of human depression.[19]

Evidence supports the possibility that acupuncture may alleviate depression through biochemical changes in the body and brain. Clinical evidence has shown significant improvement in pregnant women who used only acupuncture for the treatment of depression.[20] This is important not only because it demonstrates acupuncture's ability to treat depression, but also because it offers a non-drug alternative to women, given that anti-depressant medication in pregnancy has shown harmful effects to the fetus. It is unknown whether the particular biochemistry of depression in pregnancy is different from that of depression in other populations, possibly making acupuncture uniquely effective for this population.

Other clinical evidence has shown enhanced effects of SSRIs when acupuncture therapy is added.[21] There is also evidence of measurable depression relief in post-stroke patients, depending on factors such as time since the stroke occurred and areas of the brain affected.[22]

Biologically, depression has been associated not only with serotonin availability but also with regulation of the hypothalamic-pituitary-adrenal (HPA) axis and changes in certain brain structures. The hippocampus, a part of the brain involved in memory, has been found to shrink in size in depressed patients.[23] Other biochemical changes in depression include changes in the body's levels of dopamine, norepinephrine, GABA, glutamine, and cortisol, among others.[24] Once again, there's a cascade of physiological changes that occurs during depression, as with any disease.

Scientists haven't yet proven a one-to-one correspondence between acupuncture treatment and the repair of brain chemicals for the relief of depression. However, there is proof of acupuncture's ability to affect these neurotransmitters. In lab rats with stress-induced depression, electro-acupuncture caused an increase of serotonin receptors in the cerebral cortex.[25] In a related study, intentionally depleting serotonin eliminated the acupuncture effect of relieving depression in the animals, suggesting that acupuncture in some way enhances the availability of serotonin as part of its mechanism in relieving depression.[26] Electro-acupuncture in depressed patients has lowered abnormally elevated cortisol levels – a stress-related hormone with complex effects in the body.[27]

> *In lab rats with stress-induced depression, electro-acupuncture caused an increase of serotonin receptors in the cerebral cortex.*

In one study, scientists tested acupuncture using a known brain peptide called glial cell-derived neurotrophic factor (GDNF), which is associated with depression. They compared different treatments in three patient groups, over a six-week period:

1. Using acupoints intended to relieve depression in the first group;
2. Using acupoints *not* associated with treatment of depression in the second group;
3. Using an SSRI and no acupuncture.

They found positive responses in group (1) – using depression-related points and in group (3) – using only SSRIs with no acupuncture. These results were measured by levels of GNDF in the body and by rating patients' reported depression levels using a standardized rating scale. There was no positive response reported in group (2) – the control group using unrelated acupoints and no SSRI.

Although SSRI treatment helped relieve depression in this study, acupuncture treatment had a faster onset of action, a better response rate and a better improvement rate than the SSRI.[28]

Does it make sense to try acupuncture as a treatment approach for depression? The scientific and clinical evidence would suggest that it does. Unlike pharmaceutical medications, which have unwanted side effects, acupuncture will either help or it won't, but it can't cause harm. You can use acupuncture even if you're already using medication, and see if it causes further improvement or allows you to come off the medication and remain depression-free. In my view, there is enough evidence that acupuncture can cause regulation in brain chemistry to allow for the possibility that acupuncture's mechanism in the treatment of depression may soon be elucidated more fully.

## Anxiety

Anxiety is closely associated with depression and many people suffer from both alternately or simultaneously. Physiological changes in these two conditions seem to be related, including levels of serotonin, GABA and HPA axis hormones. In animal models for anxiety, acupuncture has induced measurable changes in levels of these neurotransmitters, just as it has in depression studies.[29]

In humans, acupuncture has been shown to improve levels of multiple

*In humans, acupuncture has been shown to improve levels of multiple anxiety-related chemicals in the body, including cortisol.[64] Imaging studies have shown that acupuncture modulates the limbic-paralimbic-neocortical network in the brain, which may mediate its anti-anxiety effects.*

anxiety-related chemicals in the body, including cortisol.[30] Imaging studies have shown that acupuncture modulates the limbic-paralimbic-neocortical network in the brain, which may mediate its anti-anxiety effects.[31]

Acupuncture is increasingly used in the treatment of veterans suffering from anxiety, PTSD, and addiction, and for addiction in the general population.[32] In these settings it is often ear acupuncture points that are used, for ease of administration and observed effectiveness, with good results reported by patients.[33]

The selection of points for human clinical trials of anxiety can vary greatly, which makes results difficult to interpret or compare. Acupuncture contends that point selection for any condition varies with the individual patient. While there are certain acupoints that are more widely used in the treatment of anxiety, the selection and combination of points in the clinic is made individually based on traditional diagnosis. Attempting to standardize the treatment by use of agreed-upon acupoints in all anxiety disorders may undermine the results of the study – if, in fact, the chosen points don't correlate well with the individual subjects.

I have treated many patients for anxiety symptoms. As with depression, multiple approaches are often beneficial, including psychotherapy and medication. Some anxiety disorders are related to trauma, some are related to exhaustion and fatigue, and others to physical injury or metabolic imbalances such as excessive thyroid activity. Anxiety disorders in women are often triggered by hormonal changes, particularly during perimenopause and menopause. In these cases, hormonal regulation through acupuncture or through hormone replacement is essential to effectively address the symptom of anxiety. This again shows the variability in causes for similar symptoms and the need for differential diagnosis that takes all the factors into account in treating anxiety.

## Insomnia

One of the most common remarks I hear from patients after their first treatment for any condition is, "I slept so well after the treatment." I recall one woman in her 60s saying that she hadn't slept at all for the last 30 years. Upon questioning, she explained that she slept just a few hours a night and only with great difficulty. Even the few hours of sleep she achieved were constantly disturbed, and she felt as if she had been awake all night. No medication helped. She came back one week after her initial acupuncture session and reported, "I slept so well all week, but I don't know if it was the acupuncture...."

Insufficient sleep has reached epidemic proportions in the United States today with as many as 70 million Americans reported to suffer from chronic insomnia. Inability to fall asleep or stay asleep leads to fatigue, a depressed immune system, mood disorders, and is associated with increased risk of serious conditions including diabetes, obesity, depression, heart attack and stroke.[34] Medications to treat insomnia have known side effects—sometimes serious, including sleepwalking, sleep-eating, or even sleep-driving.[35] A patient once told me that she'd gotten up in the night after going to sleep on an insomnia medication, and unconsciously reached for a bottle in the kitchen to quench her thirst. She drank an entire bottle of vodka, thinking it was water. That could have killed her. She only realized what had happened in the morning. It was then that she came for acupuncture to try another way to relieve her insomnia.

Evidence shows that acupuncture helps relieve insomnia.[36] As with depression and anxiety, the HPA axis and multiple neurotransmitters are involved in sleep, including norepinephrine, GABA, endogenous opiates, and melatonin, all of which are affected by acupuncture.[37]

In a clinical trial for treatment of insomnia with auricular (ear) acupressure, improvement in sleep was associated with decreased cardiac sympathetic ("fight or flight") and increased parasympathetic ("relaxation") nervous system activity.[38] This translates into calming effects. In another study, two acupoints commonly used in the treatment of insomnia patterns, HT-7 and PC-6, both located on the arm, also reduced sympathetic nervous system activity, leading to significant insomnia relief.[39]

In healthy volunteers who were not suffering from insomnia, no chemical differences were measured between the acupuncture and control groups, suggesting that the calming effect of acupuncture occurs only in symptomatic patients.[40]

GABA is a calming neurotransmitter that is found to be as much as 30 percent lower in insomnia patients than in non-symptomatic controls.[41] It is important in the regulation of sleep. Some insomnia medications are based on their ability to increase the effectiveness of GABA in the brain.[42] In studies using rat models, acupuncture has been shown to significantly increase GABA levels as well as increasing availability of its cellular receptors, which in turn makes the body better able to utilize GABA.[43] Increased GABA levels and activity in the brain are associated with sedative effects and the relief of insomnia.

GABA itself is sometimes used as a supplement to support sleep and combat anxiety. Before I had heard of its supplemental use, I saw it on the shelf in the health center where I practiced along with other health care providers. Evidently the medical doctor used it with some of his patients. I read up on it to learn more and learned that it was good for anxiety and stress, as well as insomnia. In the literature, I read that GABA supplements were not proven to cross the blood-brain barrier, and they were not expected to work for this reason. Having an experimental bent, I decided to try some myself and see if I noticed an effect. I took two capsules at around 11 a.m. and then went on with my day, forgetting that I had taken it. But within a short time, and for most of the afternoon, I felt so sleepy! I just wanted to lie down and rest, and imagined how gratifying it would be at the end of the day to go home and sleep. At around 5 p.m. I snapped out of it and felt fully awake again. That's when I recalled taking the supplement in the morning and put it together: the GABA had relaxed me to the point of somnolence. My personal research study of one convinced me that at least some GABA supplements do in fact cross the blood-brain barrier. Given my first-hand experience, I find it quite intriguing that acupuncture treatment shows a demonstrable increase in GABA availability for the relief of insomnia.

Melatonin is a more widely known supplement and a naturally occurring hormone in the body. Melatonin helps regulate the body's sleep and wake cycles. Many people have tried melatonin supplements to help them sleep, particularly when recovering from jetlag. Some people find that the supplement helps and others do not. That's because melatonin will help you sleep if your insomnia is related to a shortage of it. If it's related to something else, melatonin supplements will do nothing for you.

Studies have found reduced melatonin production in older insomnia patients.[44] Supplemental melatonin has been clinically shown to decrease the time it takes to fall asleep, increase total sleep time and improve sleep quality.[45] In a clinical acupuncture trial, melatonin secretion was significantly increased after five weeks of treatment. This increase was associated with improved sleep and reduced anxiety.[46]

Various acupuncture points may be used in the treatment of insomnia. Even with a single acupoint, such at HT-7, located on the outer wrist, a wide range of neurochemical changes associated with insomnia relief can be measured.[47] In its traditional form, acupuncture treatments involve the use of multiple acupoints at the same time. Further research may demonstrate how these combinations of acupoints work to alter a wide range of neurotransmitters simultaneously.

> *In a clinical acupuncture trial, melatonin secretion was significantly increased after five weeks of treatment. This increase was associated with improved sleep and reduced anxiety.*

## High Blood Pressure

One of every three American adults suffers from high blood pressure – also known as hypertension – a dangerous condition that increases the risk of heart attack, stroke and kidney disease.[48] In my own practice, I usually see patients who are already taking blood pressure medications by the time they seek acupuncture. I advise them to monitor their blood pressure and to keep in touch with their doctor because acupuncture commonly reduces elevated blood pressure and the medication levels have to be adjusted accordingly. My clinical experience is reflected in the results of a study that showed a significant reduction in blood pressure in patients already using hypertension medications.[49] In most cases that I have seen, patients are quickly able to reduce and then eliminate their use of blood pressure medications once they begin acupuncture treatment.

Scientific studies have confirmed that acupuncture lowers high blood pressure.[50] It has shown this effect only when specific acupoints are used.[51] Interestingly, the same points that lower high blood pressure also raise abnormally low blood pressure. Notably, these same points neither

> *Scientific studies have confirmed that acupuncture lowers high blood pressure.*

raise nor lower blood pressure in healthy individuals, but only in those whose blood pressure is abnormal.[52]

Some of the earlier research showed that acupuncture reduced myocardial ischemia, a potentially serious decrease in blood flow to the heart, when test animals were put under higher cardiac demand. Researchers found that this reduced demand for oxygen by the heart was the result of an acupuncture-induced reduction in blood pressure.[53]

Specific brain regions and nervous system pathways have been identified in the acupuncture-induced lowering of blood pressure. Opioid peptides and GABA also play a role.[54] Research continues. There is more for us to learn, yet these results confirm acupuncture's ability to regulate blood pressure and cardiovascular function, and tell us something about its mechanism.

## Acupuncture for Digestive Disorders

Acupuncture is commonly used in the treatment of various digestive problems, including acid reflux, indigestion, bloating, constipation, irritable bowel syndrome (IBS), and diarrhea. Clinical studies have begun to reveal some of the physiological effects and mechanisms by which acupuncture affects digestion. Because studies have used different acupoints with different kinds of stimulation in varying combinations, the current results don't yet form a complete explanation. However, acupuncture's effects on digestion are measurable and reproducible.

## Constipation

Constipation accounts for an estimated 8 million medical visits each year in the United States.[55] Perhaps because it is so common, the treatment of constipation with acupuncture has been the focus of quite a few research studies.

Using acupoint ST-36, traditionally prescribed to treat constipation, researchers using rat models found that it stimulates colon motility and accelerates transit time. When they inject drugs known to block specific nerve functions, the effects of the ST-36 acupuncture are blocked. This points to a sacral parasympathetic nerve pathway as the mediator of its effects on the colon.[56]

Researchers have described point-specific effects of several acupoints traditionally used in the treatment of digestive disorders.[57] While acupoint ST-36, located on the leg, increases colonic motility, acupoint ST-25, on the abdomen, slows it down. This discovery supports the traditional use of each of these points in acupuncture: ST-36 is commonly used in the treatment of constipation (to increase colonic motility); ST-25 is used to treat colitis and diarrhea (to reduce colonic activity).

> *Using acupoint ST-36, traditionally prescribed to treat constipation, researchers using rat models found that it stimulates colon motility and accelerates transit time. When they inject drugs known to block specific nerve functions, the effects of the ST-36 acupuncture are blocked.*

Clinically, acupuncture points are combined and not used in isolation. In light of this, one group of researchers tested different point combinations commonly used in acupuncture for digestion and found that electro-acupuncture of LI-11 (located at the elbow) combined with ST-37 (on the lower leg) increased motility, while electro-acupuncture of ST-25 (on the abdomen) along with ST-37 (on the lower leg) suppressed motility.[58] Here again we see point specificity with different acupuncture point combinations having different effects on colonic motility.

## Irritable Bowel Syndrome (IBS)

Irritable bowel syndrome involves pain, cramping, and disturbances including constipation and diarrhea, which often alternate. In a clinical study of IBS patients, a standard acupuncture treatment was performed using a set of five traditional acupoints, and the results were compared with another group receiving conventional medication for IBS.

The effective rate in the acupuncture group was more than 94 percent, while that of the medication group was just over 77 percent. When the patients were followed up after three months, the acupuncture group had an IBS recurrence rate much lower than that of the medication group (36.4

percent vs. 72 percent).[59] In another clinical study, one group was given acupuncture in addition to the usual medical treatment, while the other group received usual medical treatment alone. The acupuncture group did 18 percent better than the control group, and these results remained stable at six, nine, and twelve months.[60]

Patients with IBS show abnormal brain activation associated with pain perception in response to nerve signals in the digestive tract. Using functional magnetic resonance imaging (fMRI), researchers observed the brain's response to acupuncture in IBS patients.

During electro-acupuncture, increased activation was observed in several brain regions, and true acupuncture led to higher activation than sham acupuncture. Among the functions performed by these brain regions, one modulates serotonin, which has been implicated in the regulation of mood, pain and digestive function. These researchers postulate that acupuncture might reduce pain in IBS by two specific pathways: one modulating the serotonin pathway at the insula of the brain, and another modulating mood via the thalamus, a higher cortical center of the brain.[61]

In yet another study, researchers tested rats with induced diarrhea-type IBS by using medication on one group and acupuncture of two traditional acupoints, ST-36 and LV-3, on the other group. They found that IBS symptoms reduced to a significant degree in both medication and acupuncture groups compared with the control. Along with this, they found that three specific digestive hormones were lowered in both treatment groups, showing that acupuncture on its own caused the same hormonal changes as did medication, correlated with reduced IBS symptoms.[62]

## Nausea

Acupuncture is widely used to alleviate nausea. Western science has established its efficacy specifically in postoperative and chemotherapy-induced nausea.[63] Yet, clinical experience shows it to be effective for nausea from virtually any cause.

Many women in the first trimester of pregnancy get relief from nausea with acupuncture. The most extreme case of this I have ever seen was a woman with severe nausea in pregnancy that persisted well into the third trimester. Her doctors had her on a full-time intravenous pump of anti-nausea medication, and even that served only to take the edge off and reduce the frequency of vomiting. She came to try acupuncture for it. As soon as the needles were inserted, her nausea began to subside, and she had full relief from the nausea for as long as the needles were retained. I would stimulate them from time to time during her treatment, and she would stay on the table sometimes for hours and sleep, as it was the only time she could sleep without any nausea or having to get out of bed to vomit.

Scientific studies have focused on an acupoint located on the wrist, known as PC-6, traditionally used in acupuncture to treat nausea. This point also treats motion sickness. It's the same point stimulated by motion sickness-relieving wristbands that people sometimes wear when traveling.

Research studies have also tested ST-36, another point that is used clinically for nausea and vomiting. Both ST-36 and PC-6 have been shown to reduce the excessive muscle waves in the stomach that are associated with nausea.[64]

Opioids, and their receptors in the brainstem, are involved in acupuncture's anti-nausea effects in the body. When opioid receptors are blocked in that part of the brain, the anti-nausea effect of PC-6 is eliminated. This demonstrates that at least one effect of acupuncture at PC-6 is to trigger opioid release via the central nervous system.[65]

> *Both ST-36 and PC-6 have been shown to reduce the excessive muscle waves in the stomach that are associated with nausea.*

## Acupuncture in Gynecology and Fertility

Women are increasingly turning to acupuncture for gynecological concerns, including dysmenorrhea, irregular or lack of menstruation, infertility, polycystic ovarian syndrome (PCOS), pregnancy support, and to induce or support labor and childbirth.[66] There is even a treatment to help turn a fetus in breech position while still in the womb, using a point on the outside of the little toe.[67] Quite a few obstetricians now refer their patients for this treatment because it seems to work so well.

Acupuncture can also be used during labor and delivery to relieve pain, limit the use of pharmaceutical pain medication, shorter the duration of labor, and reduce the use of instrumentation, such as forceps, for delivery.[68]

Medical fertility clinics frequently provide acupuncture for patients undergoing fertility treatments such as in-vitro fertilization (IVF) and intra-uterine insemination (IUI). Although results from systematic studies have been limited, evidence suggests that using acupuncture in conjunction with embryo transfer in IVF improves rates of pregnancy and live births.[69]

Research has shown that acupuncture regulates blood flow to the uterus and ovaries. This effect appears to be mediated by the sympathetic nervous system via the brain.[70] When this is the case, it stands to reason that menstruation and fertility can be positively regulated by acupuncture. Acupuncture applied to a set of traditional points—SP-6, CV-4, CV-3 and Zigong—was shown to significantly alter hormone levels to improve endometrial receptivity in the uterus, making implantation of an embryo more likely.[71]

> *Acupuncture applied to a set of traditional points— SP-6, CV-4, CV-3 and Zigong—was shown to significantly alter hormone levels to improve endometrial receptivity in the uterus, making implantation of an embryo more likely.*

Polycystic ovarian syndrome (PCOS) is a disorder commonly causing infertility in women. It is associated with irregular ovulation and with metabolic symptoms including insulin resistance, abdominal obesity, hypertension, and excessive androgen production, causing excess body and facial hair growth, among other things.

PCOS provides a good model for testing the effects of acupuncture on the female reproductive system, while offering insight into how acupuncture might specifically help PCOS patients to conceive. In studies of women with the syndrome, low frequency electro-acupuncture treatments were shown to have long lasting effects on regulating ovulation as well as on the metabolic symptoms, including insulin resistance. Using acupoints BL-23, BL-28 and SP-9 induced an increase in ovulation along with improved levels of reproductive hormones including LH (luteinizing hormone), FSH (follicle stimulating hormone), testosterone and beta-endorphins.[72]

Acupuncture studies using rats with PCOS demonstrated that low-frequency electro-acupuncture reduced insulin resistance and regulated several hormones associated with sympathetic nervous system function.[73]

In a study of women with primary ovarian insufficiency, the use of traditional acupoints increased estrogen levels and decreased follicle-stimulating hormone (FSH) and luteinizing hormone (LH) levels, leading to the restoration of regular menstruation while reducing hot flashes and night sweats. These results remained stable during the three-month follow-up period. Researchers found that acupuncture produced both central and peripheral effects. The central effect worked via the hypothalamus in the brain to alter hormone levels. The peripheral effect worked through the spinal segment at the level of the ovaries. Both central and peripheral effects influenced sympathetic nervous system activity with an end result of normalizing ovulation and improving fertility.[74]

## Acupuncture in Support of Neurogenesis in the Brain: Parkinson's Disease, Stroke, Alzheimer's Disease

Some of the most challenging medical cases involve nerve damage and dysfunction in the brain, including Parkinson's and Alzheimer's diseases, as well as post-stroke effects. The entire question of whether acupuncture can promote restoration of brain function or healing of brain or nerve cells in general is one that researchers want to answer. Specifically, they want to know if acupuncture can improve brain function in any of these serious diseases.

Science used to believe that adult nerve regeneration (neurogenesis) was impossible. Research has since shown that new nerve stem cells are generated throughout life and mature into functional nerve and brain cells. Nerve cell development increases in parts of the brain after stroke and in Alzheimer's patients, as the brain presumably attempts to compensate for lost function in other brain cells due to damage or disease.[75]

Both improving the nutritional environment and adding physical exercise are shown to promote adult nerve growth. Current research is showing how electro-stimulation can be used to stimulate new pathways and enhanced function in the brain, leading to dramatically reduced symptoms in intractable conditions like Parkinson's Disease and Multiple Sclerosis.[76]

There is evidence to suggest that acupuncture is another approach that supports increased nerve growth in adults. Several studies suggest that acupuncture causes increased production of nerve growth factors, which may be responsible for generating new nerve cell growth, although its precise mechanism is not yet fully known.[77]

*Several studies suggest that acupuncture causes increased production of nerve growth factors, which may be responsible for generating new nerve cell growth, although its precise mechanism is not yet fully known.*

Clinically, using acupuncture for patients with Parkinson's Disease has shown mixed results and has not provided any conclusive evidence that it can improve the condition.[78]

Animal studies have provided opportunities for more specific measurements and have shown improvements in motor function correlated with measurable neuronal changes in the brain.[79] Acupuncture triggers the activation of specific brain regions, correlating with these motor improvements. We know from multiple studies that acupuncture modulates release and activity of hormones, neurotransmitters, transcription factors, endogenous opioids, and specific brain regions, depending on the acupoints selected and the type of stimulation used. Since Parkinson's Disease is associated in part with altered dopamine levels, it is natural to look for acupoints that modulate dopamine generation and that influence the part of the brain involved in this process, in addition to improving motor functions. In one study using a mouse model of Parkinson's Disease, stimulating acupoint GB-34 enhanced synaptic dopamine availability, resulting in improved motor function.[80]

*In one study using a mouse model of Parkinson's Disease, stimulating acupoint GB-34 enhanced synaptic dopamine availability, resulting in improved motor function.*

Studies using acupuncture for the treatment of stroke-related symptoms as well as other brain diseases are under way. Using rat models, electro-acupuncture at acupoints ST-36 and LI-11 significantly reduced neurological deficits and cerebral infarction (tissue death due to a lack of oxygen). Acupuncture was found to increase levels of chemicals that stimulate cerebral cell proliferation, thereby inducing brain repair after stroke injury. This study showed not only that acupuncture had a neuroprotective effect in ischemic stroke, but it may exert these effects by activating a specific biochemical pathway for cellular regeneration.[81]

In a study of mild cognitive impairment due to Alzheimer's Disease, researchers used acupoints LI-4 and LV-3 on diagnosed patients and healthy control subjects. Functional MRI (fMRI) data showed altered brain activity in the temporal and frontal lobes of the brain in the patient group, in regions closely related to memory and cognition. The healthy subjects showed no change in brain activity, suggesting these effects were activated only when the brain function was impaired.[82]

In my own clinical experience I have seen definite improvement using acupuncture in stroke patients, with faster and more complete recovery the sooner acupuncture is started post-stroke. Recovery is also better in younger patients. I have not seen good clinical results in Parkinson's patients, but I have encountered acupuncturists who believe they are able to arrest symptom development, particularly through scalp acupuncture techniques. I haven't heard of measurable improvement in Alzheimer's patients as a result of acupuncture treatment, nor have I treated many patients suffering from the disease.

Acupuncture has been extensively used in China for the treatment of cognitive impairment from stroke. Treatment of Alzheimer's Disease has not been as extensively reported there. Suggestive evidence supports further inquiry, but there is as yet insufficient data to draw firm conclusions about how well acupuncture works in these cases, by what mechanisms it may be working, or in which subtypes of diseases it may be effective.

## Treating Diabetes with Acupuncture

There are two types of diabetes: type 1 and type 2. Type 1 is also known as juvenile-onset diabetes and is caused when the immune system attacks the pancreas, wiping out its ability to produce insulin.

By contrast, type 2, also known as adult-onset diabetes, occurs in the vast majority of diabetes patients and is associated with insulin resistance – an inability to use the body's insulin – which is frequently brought on in part by an improper diet.

Once insulin resistance sets in, the body is unable to use its own insulin. Blood sugar then becomes excessively elevated, because it's the job of insulin to move sugars from the blood into the cells to use as fuel. The sugar is then converted to fat by the liver, causing excess weight gain and obesity.

Other risks associated with type 2 diabetes include stroke, heart disease, kidney disease, and circulatory problems that can lead to amputation in extreme cases. Acupuncture has been studied for use in type 2 diabetes patients to determine its effects in controlling blood sugar and restoring normal insulin sensitivity in patients.[83]

In one human study, acupuncture produced a reduction in blood sugar and body weight compared with the control group. Researchers found that acupuncture stimulated an increase in serum insulin and C-peptide levels, leading to lower blood sugar. These results occurred in obese but non-diabetic volunteers without insulin resistance.[84]

In another study using diabetic rats, researchers showed that one subtype of endorphin, triggered by acupuncture, was involved in mediating lowered blood sugar levels. They were able to do this by first doing acupuncture and showing that it lowered blood sugar levels. Then they administered an opiate antagonist (endorphins are a form of natural opiates secreted in the body) and found that this blocked acupuncture's blood sugar lowering effects.[85]

Other studies using diabetic rats have shown that acupuncture improved insulin sensitivity, increased insulin blood levels, and lowered blood sugar.[86]

Through these studies, acupuncture has been shown to regulate blood sugar levels in type 2 diabetes. Measurable effects include increased insulin levels and insulin sensitivity, reduced insulin resistance, and release of endorphins that regulate blood sugar levels.

Research evidence suggests that acupuncture points exert some of their effects via the brain and the spinal cord, and others through the endocrine system.

# Key Points

- Scientific research has demonstrated proven effects of acupuncture in the body.
- Science uses three main research approaches: *basic research* takes measurements on human and animal subjects in the laboratory; *randomized controlled trials* test healthy or symptomatic human volunteers clinically to measure acupuncture's effects; and *systematic reviews* combine multiple studies to establish trends and to make broad statements about acupuncture's effectiveness.
- Acupuncture triggers diverse biological processes, including the production and secretion of active chemicals, including DNA transcription.[87]
- Acupuncture induces release of endorphins, the body's natural painkillers, as well as natural anti-inflammatory substances, among others.
- Acupuncture's pain relieving actions are found to work through at least two different pathways, affecting both the nervous system and the hormonal system.
- Some acupoints seem to affect body regions innervated by the same spinal nerve root, while others affect seemingly unrelated areas.
- Acupuncture's effects vary by which point is used and by how the needle is stimulated, manually or with electro-stimulation of different frequencies.
- Brain scans show that acupuncture signals reach the brain and affect multiple regions, depending on which points are used.
- Research has proven measurable effects of acupuncture in the treatment of pain conditions including lower back pain, carpal tunnel syndrome and neuropathic pain syndromes.

- Science has documented specific, reproducible, relevant physiological effects using acupuncture in the treatment of depression, anxiety, insomnia, high blood pressure, constipation, irritable bowel syndrome (IBS), nausea, gynecology and fertility, and diabetes.
- Acupuncture on brain-related diseases is ongoing and has shown measurable effects on growth factors, brain activity, and motor function.

## CHAPTER SIX

# How Does Acupuncture Really Work?

"The difficulty lies not so much in developing
new ideas as in escaping from old ones."
- John Maynard Keynes

Science has proven that acupuncture has measurable therapeutic effects in the body. A fundamental question remains: what is the mechanism by which acupuncture needling produces these effects? More specifically, what is the "anatomy" of an acupuncture point or meridian? Exactly how does an acupuncture needle trigger nervous system and hormonal signals? How does it send messages to the brain and cause system-wide healing effects? Why do acupoints in different locations have different effects in the body?

Though we don't yet know definitively, there is an increasing amount of scientific research suggesting that fascia, our connective tissue, may provide one clue to the answer. I'm going to share with you some of the research that I find most intriguing, and how it might relate to acupuncture's ancient theoretical concepts of meridians and acupoints. This is a journey of possibilities and not settled science. To use existing data to imagine possibilities is the essence of the scientific approach.

## The Acupuncture Mystery: Beyond the Nervous System

We tend to think of the nervous system as the main unifying network in the body. From the brain, through the spine, reaching into every limb and organ, the nervous system senses and responds to our inner and outer environment. Through our own experience we know that needling, like any stimulation to the skin, reaches the brain – we can feel it. Therefore, much of the acupuncture research has focused on nervous system effects. However, nerves on their own cannot provide a full explanation of acupuncture's actions.

When an acupoint is treated with needling – or with pressure or heat for that matter – various protective and homeostatic events are set in motion. Chemicals and hormones – anti-pain, pro-inflammatory (inflammation is part of the body's initial healing response), immune and tissue repairing substances – are secreted directly into the area by local cells. Nerves are triggered that send messages to the spinal cord and brain.

Acupuncture activates multiple self-regulating systems that work together in a non-linear, coordinated way to protect, heal, and maintain the body's integrity. Connective tissue, as it turns out, is also activated by acupuncture to produce both local and far-reaching effects.[1]

Let's take a look at the interconnected web of connective tissue and see how it might relate to acupuncture's web of meridians.

## The Interconnected Web of Acupuncture Anatomy: Jing Luo

The mysterious acupuncture meridians have not yet been found anatomically. Or have they? The ancient Chinese described acupuncture meridians as a web of interconnecting vessels which they called *jing luo*. This term, *jing luo*, is variously and imperfectly translated into English as meridians, vessels, channels and collaterals, channels and connecting channels, conduits and network vessels.[2]

The visual depiction of *jing luo* appears like a web and evokes the image of a three dimensional woven fabric, with *jing* forming the vertical threads and *luo* the horizontal threads. In fact the modern Chinese term for the internet is *wang luo*, "global interconnected web." The *jing luo* travel vertically from head to toe and horizontally between exterior and interior, linking the surface of the body to the internal organs and cells, and all parts of the body to all other parts.

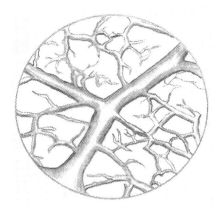

Acupuncture meridians form a web of interconnecting vessels that permeate the body three-dimensionally. In acupuncture they are called "jing luo."

It is through the *jing luo* that *qi* is said to travel, and acupuncture points are located along its pathways. Stimulating acupuncture points with needles, heat, pressure, or even laser light causes changes in the flow of *qi* along the *jing luo*, affecting the function of tissues both near and far from the point. What could possibly respond in this way and extend so far?

## The Interconnected Web of Western Anatomy: Fascia

The fascial connective tissue constitutes a whole-body regulatory system all its own, one that interconnects with every other part of the body. It surrounds and interpenetrates every organ, muscle, bone, vessel and cell.

Fascia is one of several forms of connective tissue. It is more pervasive than the nervous system or blood vessels (although blood vessels are themselves a form of connective tissue, and nerves are covered with it as well). Through contiguous sheaths that branch into finer filaments wrapping and connecting with organs and cells, fascia holds us together and keeps everything in its proper place. It can be visualized as a kind of "bubble wrap" that creates distinct regions and pockets in which organs, bones, nerves, and all our cells are held in place. Not only does it wrap and contain these structures, but it threads right into them. If you were to remove everything but the fascia what would remain is a perfect replica of the body itself. No other system does that. And yet, I never learned much about it in anatomy class. You probably didn't either.

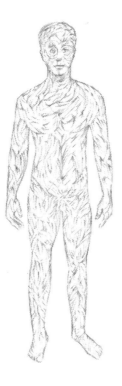

The web of connective tissue known as fascia is like a three-dimensional fabric that wraps, interpenetrates and connects every organ and tissue in the body.

Although the fascial web is the single most pervasive system in the body, until recently fascia has been almost completely overlooked in medicine. The superficial fascia is peeled away when dissecting cadavers, as though it were a mere sheath with no function. As it turns out, its state of health is intimately related to our health and disease. In addition to providing structure, fascia is like a three dimensional fabric through which internal messages in the body can be transmitted over long distances.

Through stress, injury and inflammation the fascia can become firm and solid, also known as fibrotic, instead of soft and pliable. You end up with a hard webbing enclosing and interpenetrating vital body parts and essentially strangling them – restricting movement of organs and muscles, causing pain and dysfunction – and even abnormal tissue growth – while keeping blood and nerve supply from reaching their targets. Scarring is one example of this effect, which we can see when it occurs on the skin's surface.

The same process occurs inside the body not only from incisions, tears and surgery but also from overuse, as in carpal tunnel syndrome or frozen shoulder. It can occur in blood vessels, leading to high blood pressure; in the feet causing plantar fasciitis, making walking painful; in the bladder causing urinary frequency or recurring infections; or in the lungs, creating breathing problems.

> *Fascial restrictions can transmit signals all the way into cells, affecting gene expression, alternately blocking or stimulating secretion of hormones, neurotransmitters and otherwise changing our biochemistry and physiology. These events, in turn, can contribute to disease or to healing.*

Fascial restrictions can transmit signals all the way into cells, affecting gene expression, alternately blocking or stimulating secretion of hormones, neurotransmitters and otherwise changing our biochemistry and physiology.[3] These events, in turn, can contribute to disease or to healing.

In addition, because of the fascia's pervasive connections, restrictions in one area can be transmitted to other parts of the body, causing imbalance, pain and dysfunction.

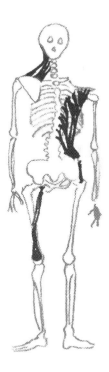

Fascial restrictions that start in the neck and shoulder can lead to restricted fascia in the hip and leg, causing widespread structural imbalance and pain.

In this illustration you can see how a pattern of tension which may have started in the neck and shoulder is transmitted to the hip and leg through fascial restrictions. This patient may experience hip pain, not realizing that his neck tension plays into the problem. Relieving his hip pain may require releasing the fascial restrictions in the neck as well for lasting relief.

## Fascia's Integrative Function

If you could look under the skin at a microscopic level, you would see pervasive fascial filaments comprised of elastin and collagen, surrounded by a semi-fluid extracellular matrix. This matrix is a gel-like substance consisting of water containing specialized carbohydrate and protein molecules known as glycosaminoglycans, glycoproteins, and glucoaminoglycans.[4] Often referred to as "ground substance," it allows the elastin and collagen fibers to glide and move, supporting the health of all the body's tissues as well as our flexibility and movement.[5] It carries nutrients to cells and waste products away from them. Found within the extracellular matrix are fibroblasts, connective tissue cells that both generate the ground substance in which they reside and respond to its signals.[6]

Fascia is characterized by plasticity and an ability to remodel itself in response to mechanical stress.[7] Elastin confers its ability to stretch while collagen confers structure and resilience. Loss of collagen in the skin as we age is responsible for reduced tone leading to wrinkles.

Mechanical signals – from pressure, pulling, injury, or repetitive strain – are picked up by the fascia and transmitted to other parts of the body in a process known as *mechanotransduction*.[8] Mechanotransduction simply means that pressure (or needling) creates a signal that is carried to other parts of the body. A very simple analogy might be turning a lever to open or close a window. Movement in one location creates changes someplace else.

When a mechanical signal is introduced, whether through prolonged stretch or acupuncture stimulation, it is converted into electrical and biochemical changes that have measurable physiological effects. Stimulated fibroblasts release ATP (adenosine triphosphate) into the extracellular environment. Inside of our cells ATP is known for its function as fuel. Outside of the cells, ATP can be converted into adenosine, which can act as a local painkiller, providing another possible mechanism for acupuncture pain relief.[9]

These fibroblasts also begin to reorganize their internal structure and change shape, initiating extensive and far-reaching relaxation of the connective tissue. Cells throughout the body are capable of picking up mechanically-induced signals, conveyed by fascia, and converting them into physiological responses, including changes in genetic expression. This is mediated by specialized molecules embedded in the cell membrane. Known as integrins, these molecules connect and communicate with an organized network of microfilaments within the cell that make up the cytoskeleton, its internal structure. In this way, cellular responses can occur far from the original stimulation, in regions that are not connected by nervous system pathways, reaching all the way to the nucleus of these distant cells where gene activity is controlled.

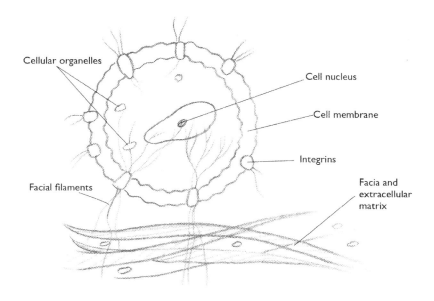

Fascial filaments pass through the cell membrane via specialized molecules known as integrins, reaching all the way into the nucleus of the cell. In this way, mechanical signals can induce cellular responses, including DNA transcription, in locations far from the original stimulus. This may be part of how acupuncture exerts its effects, via mechanical signals that move from the site of the acupuncture needle to other parts of the body.

Mechanical signals working through the fascia act extremely rapidly, moving at about 30 meters per second, about 30 million times faster than chemical signals.[10] (By comparison, nerve signals move at rates between 30 and 100 meters per second.) There is intriguing evidence that cells may also communicate through piezoelectricity – electromagnetic signals induced by pressure – as well as through biophotonic information, which is capable of moving throughout the body at the speed of light.[11]

It is becoming clear that there are multiple communication pathways integrating the body simultaneously, not all of which are as yet understood. One specialized aspect of the fascial system is the perineural connective tissue, which covers nerves and conveys signals of its own. Together, the nerves and the perineural connective tissue have been referred to as the "dual nervous system."[12] While nerves are designed to direct their signals to and from very precise locations, the perineural tissue is believed to send diffuse electromagnetic signals throughout the body, thereby exerting an integrative function. This raises the intriguing possibility that at least one aspect of what the ancient Chinese called "*qi*" may be electromagnetic in nature.

## How Acupuncture Describes Fascia

The ancient Chinese acupuncturists may well have recognized the network of fascia that filled the spaces between the organs and tissues of the body. Aspects of this network and its functions are described in early acupuncture texts in terms of membranes (*huang*), fat (*gao*), cavities and texture (*cou li*) and also by the Triple Heater, an "organ" in its own right with its own meridian system that corresponds to no known organ in Western anatomy.

Contemporary Chinese medicine scholar and clinician Giovanni Maciocia explains that the membranes (*huang*) "are the connective tissue that fills the abdominal cavity and surrounds the organs...."[13] The Triple Heater is, among other things, a system of body cavities, including the chest, abdomen and pelvis, traditionally seen as the three "heaters" or "burning spaces," as well as all other cavities and spaces in joints and between body tissues.[14] In keeping with Chinese medicine's inclination to focus on function and physiology over form and anatomy, the Triple Heater as an "organ" serves to control all the cavities, the movement of fluids that irrigate them, and the movement of *qi* in and out of them.

Within and amongst these ancient acupuncture concepts we can find elements of the fascial system as we know it, and its functions as we are coming to understand them. As we see over and again, acupuncture's concepts of anatomy and physiology don't readily translate into Western anatomy and physiology in a one to one correspondence. Instead, we find that the body is viewed and described through a different lens in which some functions are grouped together and others are separated in ways that differ from how we describe them. Nevertheless, we can see that the concept of fascia and its physiological functions were quite likely understood by ancient Chinese acupuncturists and built in to the system of diagnosis and treatment.

## Connecting Outside to Inside: Meridian Palpation and Acupoint Location

A key element in traditional acupuncture diagnosis involves palpation of meridians. The qualities felt in the skin, muscles, and connective tissue along meridian pathways provide information about the status of the internal organs and overall balance in the body.

Another way of saying this is that internal health or imbalance can be observed and felt on the surface of the body. Meridian palpation reveals qualities such as elasticity, tenderness, softness, puffiness, firmness, knottiness, or nodules. Each of these qualities reflects something about the health of the meridian and its associated organ system.

Similarly, palpation is used when selecting and locating acupuncture points for treatment. Acupuncturists follow anatomical guidelines to approach the acupuncture point, but its precise location is determined by feeling for it. It may be felt as a "hole" or a softness, or alternatively at times as a nodule or firmness. When an organ and its associated meridian system need balancing, acupuncture points display distinct qualities of softness, firmness or tenderness that would not otherwise be found in a healthy patient. In the patient, these points will often evoke greater tenderness.

> *When an organ and its associated meridian system need balancing, acupuncture points display distinct qualities of softness, firmness or tenderness that would not otherwise be found in a healthy patient.*

When we think in terms of fascia it gives us a way to understand these palpable qualities in meridians and acupuncture points. The fascia in health is known to provide the body with a healthy tone – flexibility within structure, not too tense and not too soft. But when diseased, injured or otherwise altered it may exhibit excess tension or flaccidity. Because the fascia interpenetrates and connects wide-ranging regions of the body, a dysfunction in an internal organ can be conveyed through fascia to the surface of the body, even at some distance away. Likewise, by the same mechanisms, an injury on the surface of the body may affect the health of internal organs.[15]

This aspect of point location and selection of "active" acupoints for treatment presents a significant challenge for evidence-based clinical acupuncture trials. For the purposes of scientific method and controls, groups of patients are treated using predetermined points and the effects of those treatments are measured and compared. However, even patients suffering from the same complaint, such as back pain, arthritis or hypertension, might be treated differently using traditional acupuncture. The same symptoms may be seen to arise from different root causes, and that determines acupoint selection. Patients with different root causes for the same symptom might not have the same active acupuncture points. In light of this, using a standard set of acupoints based on symptoms alone may not yield reliable scientific data. Unless an assessment of the patient's individual condition is included in clinical studies along with acupoint location through palpation, the research may not provide accurate results.

## Acupoint Anatomy: What's in an Acupuncture Point?

What is the anatomy of an acupuncture point? What distinguishes acupoints from non-acupoints? And what actually happens when an acupuncture needle is inserted and stimulated either manually or with electricity? This is of particular relevance when non-acupoints are used as controls in clinical acupuncture studies.

Sham acupuncture, as it is called, is the use of non-acupuncture points to compare their effects to true acupuncture points. Results often demonstrate that sham acupuncture can produce measurable physiological effects, though often less pronounced than those produced by true acupuncture points. This causes scientists to scratch their heads and wonder if sham points can be considered valid neutral controls, especially since they don't yet know what constitutes a true acupuncture point. And skeptics point to this as "proof" that acupuncture points and meridians are illusory imaginings of the ancient Chinese mind.

When acupuncture needles are inserted, they are rotated to induce a characteristic "needle grasp" that can be felt by the practitioner. Patients may feel this as a sensation of aching, soreness or pressure, known as "*de qi*," and they may also notice a propagated sensation that feels something like a momentary electrical current traveling along a trajectory. Patients can describe precisely where they feel this moving sensation, and in doing so they are usually describing the textbook pathway of the acupuncture meridian, even without knowing anything about these pathways.

Although it may feel like a nerve has been touched, perceived and actual meridian pathways don't generally follow the course of major nerves. Instead, it is thought that acupuncture needles may create a mechanical signal through the connective tissue.[16] This, in turn, activates multiple types of afferent nerves sending messages to the brain while also inducing other physical responses directly through mechanotransduction.

Dr. Helene Langevin is a research physician who has been one of the key figures leading the research into the relationship between acupuncture and fascia. Dr. Langevin and her colleagues have been able to show that when acupuncture needles are inserted and rotated to induce the characteristic "needle grasp," connective tissue winds around the needle, initiating a mechanical pull into the tissue. In turn, this induces changes in fibroblasts that create further pulling of connective tissue fibers, sending a wave of contraction and cellular activation that may explain the propagated sensation often felt by patients.[17]

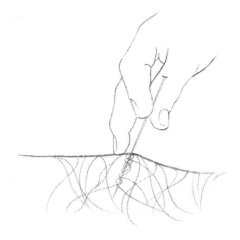

Connective tissue winds around the acupuncture needle,
sending a mechanically-induced wave of contraction and cellular
activation that may help explain how acupuncture works.

When researchers compared needle grasp in acupuncture and non-acupuncture points, they found it common to both, but significantly greater in force at acupuncture points.[18] They further found that acupuncture meridians are mostly located along fascial planes – areas where large sheaths of fascia line up – between muscles or between the muscle and bone or tendon.

Fascial planes contain much greater amounts of connective tissue. This could explain why acupuncture points inserted along meridians would display greater needle grasp than non-acupuncture points inserted into regions with less connective tissue. Since the signal transduction through connective tissue has been shown to exert far-reaching effects, including nervous system triggering, it follows that non-acupuncture points would have measurable but less pronounced effects than acupuncture points.[19]

Research has suggested that acupuncture meridians might be associated with increased electrical conductivity, but the findings have been equivocal. The way that conductivity is measured scientifically is by impedance – the degree to which a signal is impeded or slowed down. One group of researchers measured electrical impedance along meridians in relation to the fascial tissue density. They reasoned that if acupuncture meridians are associated with increased connective tissue, and if that connective tissue conducts electrical charge better, this might provide more insight into the anatomical basis for acupuncture meridians and their physiology.

This research revealed reduced impedance along the Large Intestine meridian on the arm compared with an adjacent control location. Yet in the other two meridians they tested – the Liver and Bladder meridians – both on the leg, there was no significant difference found.

However, what's most interesting is this: they also found an increased density of collagenous tissue along the Large Intestine meridian compared with its adjacent control area and with the meridians on the leg.[20] This result suggests that reduced impedance – and increased electrical conductivity – may be related to the density of collagenous fibers and their unique bioelectrical properties. We would then have to ask why this property is found in some acupuncture meridians but not in others. Increased electrical conductivity may be but one of several properties that define a meridian and its functions.

This evidence suggests that acupuncture may primarily affect the fascial system, which in turn triggers nervous system, circulatory and hormonal responses, and that all of these combine to produce measurable healing effects. If this is the case, it is not one linear mechanism that will explain acupuncture's effects, but a concert of responses working simultaneously and in harmony, perhaps synergistically.

Scientific evidence of acupoints and meridians is increasingly showing a relationship to the fascial web interconnecting all parts of the body. As research continues, we may just come to find that the ancient Chinese acupuncturists of two thousand years ago, using their own observations and perceptions, understood the fascial system even better than we do today. Perhaps they called it *jing luo*, *cou li*, *huang* and Triple Heater, and treated it using needles, pressure and heat to cause whole-body targeted healing effects.

## The Body's Elegant Design: Tensegrity

To better understand how a small imbalance, repetitive strain, or old injury can lead to pain or disease in other parts of the body, often much later, it is helpful to understand the concept of tensegrity.

Tensegrity is a term coined by the architect Buckminster Fuller to describe a structural design based on "tensional integrity." In architecture, tensegrity takes many forms, one of which is the geodesic dome. Its structure is supported by the assembly of isolated components in compression held within a net of continuous tension. It confers the ability to yield without breaking. Tensegrity structures confer increased structural resilience, minimize the material required, and organize space in the most efficient way possible.

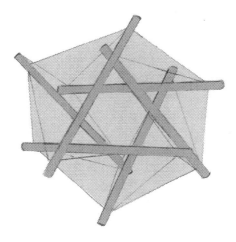

A tensegrity structure is supported by the assembly of isolated components in compression held within a net of continuous tension. It confers the ability to yield without breaking.

Physician and researcher Donald E. Ingber of Harvard Medical School has described tensegrity as "the architecture of life." Dr. Ingber's pioneering work in bioengineering led him to the discovery that the human body is itself organized by tensegrity, supported by the union of tensioned and compressed components. On the gross structural level, the muscles and connective tissues provide continuous pull while the bones provide discontinuous compression. As you move into smaller and smaller systems in the body, tensegrity continues to organize all of its structures down to the cellular, molecular and genetic levels. The body's tensegrity-based design confers maximum strength and resilience, stabilizing its shape and integrating structure and function within and between all levels.[21]

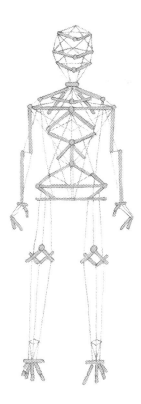

The human body's tensegrity-based design confers maximum
strength and resilience, stabilizing its shape and integrating
structure and function within and between all levels.

Tensegrity within the fascial system has been captured in videos
taken by Dr. Jean Claude Guimberteau, a French hand surgeon, on
living tissue.[22] This and other research shows tensegrity-based movement
and resilience made possible by healthy, flexible fascia, and how that
movement is impeded when the semi-fluid environment hardens due to
trauma, strain, injury, and unresolved inflammation. This is important in
understanding how injury and illness can cause wide-ranging disorder in
the body. Fibrotic fascia impedes circulation and movement at the site of
injury as well as in regions connected to it by fascial tissue. It also helps
us understand how the system of acupuncture might work through the
fascia to heal.

# The Placebo Effect: Mind as Healer

In considering acupuncture's mechanism, let's take a moment to talk about the placebo effect and its role in acupuncture healing. Among the questions raised about acupuncture is whether it is working solely due to the patient's expectation of recovery: the placebo effect.

It is widely accepted that a patient's expectation can produce measurable therapeutic changes. In scientific studies of acupuncture, as in all scientific research, great effort is made to control for this. To prove whether a drug or other medical intervention works, scientists attempt to separate the effects of expectation from those attributable solely to the treatment being tested. The double-blind randomized controlled trial (RCT) is the ultimate expression of this. In this type of study, patients are randomly assigned and neither doctor nor patient knows whether a medication being given is real or not.

In acupuncture trials this is particularly challenging because it is virtually impossible to administer clinical treatments without the provider knowing whether a true or sham acupoint is being used. Attempts to control for the placebo effect in acupuncture clinical studies include treatment of non-acupoints for comparison of results and ensuring that there is minimal interaction between patient and acupuncturist.

There is enough well-controlled scientific data by now to conclude that acupuncture's effects are not solely due to placebo effects. Much of this data has been gathered in studies using animal models. It is safe to assume that lab rats haven't read or heard anything that would make them anticipate acupuncture's effectiveness. You might say that simply handling the animal could produce these effects, apart from the acupuncture, but even this has been controlled for in lab studies. Similarly, cuddling a baby doesn't make his fever go away.

> *There is enough well-controlled scientific data by now to conclude that acupuncture's effects are not solely due to placebo effects.*

But within a few minutes of acupuncture treatment you can observe the physical changes right before your eyes, as the baby's color changes, his agitation decreases, and his fever goes down.

While it is standard in scientific research to control for the placebo effect, clinically we are wise to use it as part of the treatment. Placebo effect is not something fake; it is real medicine in its own right. It is using the power of the mind for healing. The mind's healing power is so great that we strive and struggle to eliminate it in our scientific validation of medical interventions.

Ethical concerns in biomedicine get in the way of using placebo treatment. While studies have frequently shown placebo pills to be as effective as anti-depressant drugs, for example, it's an ethical dilemma for the doctor who can't surreptitiously administer an inert pill to the patient in place of the drug he says he's providing. Doctors can't go through the motions of providing a surgical fix to the patient's knee without actually doing it, though in some cases this might be just as effective in healing.[23] What doctors can do, however, is to support the patient with encouragement and engage the mind's healing power with each treatment they provide.

In the acupuncture clinic, I use the placebo effect in every treatment, and consider this part of what makes it potent. I actively seek to engage the patient's self-healing abilities. I'm well aware that part of what helps patients recover comes through the interaction itself. Just by listening, affirming someone's experience, touching their pain, self-healing forces within the patient are stimulated. By demonstrating for the patient how a particular acupuncture point immediately relieves a specific area of tension or pain, she gains confidence in the treatment causing her own mind's healing power to interpret the entire treatment as healing – thereby making it more so. By informing a patient while inserting a needle in a point, "This point is very effective in relieving headache," I'm focusing the patient's mind to call forth its ability to enhance its effect.

Far from being something to eliminate, placebo is one of the tools used in clinical acupuncture treatment to increase its effectiveness. We intentionally augment acupuncture's inherent healing effects by engaging the healing abilities of the patient's own mind-body connection.

# Key Points

- In addition to the nervous system, brain, and hormones, acupuncture activates part of the body's connective tissue known as fascia.
- The acupuncture meridian system, known as "jing luo" appears like a web that moves throughout the body in the same way as fascia.
- Fascia, made up of largely elastin and collagen, is more pervasive than any other system in the body, enclosing and interpenetrating all other cells, organs and tissues.
- Through stress, injury and inflammation the fascia can become firm and solid, instead of soft and pliable, causing pain and dysfunction.
- Mechanical signals — from pressure, pulling, injury or strain — can be transmitted by fascia to other parts of the body through a process known as mechanotransduction.
- Cells throughout the body pick up mechanical signals in the fascia and convert them into physiological responses, including changes in genetic expression, through specialized molecules in the cell membrane known as integrins.
- Integrins in the cell membrane, when stimulated by fascial signals, communicate with a network of filaments within the cell, sending messages to cellular structures, including the nucleus and its DNA.
- Mechanical signals working through the fascia act rapidly, about 30 million times faster than chemical signals. Cells may also communicate through electromagnetic signals induced by pressure (piezoelectricity) and through biophotonic information, which is capable of moving through the body at the speed of light.
- Acupuncture points on the body frequently correspond to areas of greater density of fascial connective tissue, while acupuncture's meridians correlate closely with known fascial planes.

- Acupuncture needling creates measurable changes in connective tissue, conducting mechanical signals some distance away from the point.
- The entire body structure is based on tensegrity, helping to explain how the network of fascia can receive and convey signals throughout the body.
- In research, scientists attempt to eliminate the placebo effect, the tendency for patients to improve in response to their expectations of recovery; it is controlled in acupuncture studies as well. In clinical acupuncture practice, the placebo effect is understood as the mind's power to heal, can be used to enhance the treatment outcomes.

# CHAPTER SEVEN

· · · · · · · · · · · · · · · · · · · · · ·

# How to Use Acupuncture for Your Health

"You never change things by fighting the existing reality.
To change something, build a new model that
makes the existing model obsolete."
—Buckminster Fuller

The human body possesses innate self-healing abilities. When you catch a cold or flu, your immune system kicks in to fight it off and you recover. When you cut your finger, that too heals: a scab forms and the skin repairs itself. When you get a sunburn, it heals, and if you have fair skin then you may tan – your body's way of protecting you from further sunburns.

Broken bones, when properly reset, go on to mend themselves. Even cancer cells – science tells us – arise with regularity in our bodies when individual cells go awry, and are controlled by our immune system – up to a point. The same interconnecting systems that serve to integrate the body and maintain health can cause pain and illness when they break down.

Trauma, illness and injury can overwhelm the body's self-healing abilities. When that happens, we end up with conditions like chronic inflammation, adhesive scars, thickening of bone, muscle or connective tissue, and even cancerous growth. These in turn lead to pain, dysfunction, and disease. Conversely, when the offending injury is relieved and therapeutic treatment is given early enough, the body has the capacity to reverse the damage and to heal.

Acupuncture engages the self-regulatory systems that are designed to help the body heal and repair. It serves to remove blockages and restore the body's healthy function. It's not acupuncture that heals, but your own body. Acupuncture simply activates and supports your own body's healing functions and *you* do the healing.

## Holistic Health: Western and Complementary Medicine Combined

A patient with breast cancer can't use acupuncture to treat it. She needs conventional medical treatment – surgery and possibly chemotherapy or radiation. So she goes in for a mastectomy and comes out with pain and stiffness – that last *forever* – around her chest and upper back. She is exhausted, her adrenals are weak and tired, and her body is dealing with the after-effects of surgery, chemotherapy and other medications. Once she is cancer-free, her physicians discharge her and nothing else is done to help put her back together again. This is the time for her to get acupuncture. (Acupuncture can also be used during chemotherapy to help alleviate the side effects, including nausea.)

Without any adjunct treatment, in addition to unrelenting chest tension and pain, this patient will often drag herself along for years in a state of exhaustion that leads to depression, and later come down with other ailments from a weakened immune system, unresolved inflammation, and a body that has lost its functional integrity. In her case, combining conventional medical treatment – scans, surgery, chemotherapy – with complementary care – acupuncture, manual therapy, nutrition, and herbal medicine – constitutes holistic medicine. It's taking the best of what each has to offer and using them together.

The World Health Organization defines holistic health as: "Viewing man in his totality within a wide ecological spectrum, and…. emphasizing the view that ill health or disease is brought about by an imbalance, or disequilibrium, of man in his total ecological system and not only by the causative agent and pathogenic evolution."[1]

By this definition, "holistic" health involves physical, mental, emotional, and spiritual well-being that takes our whole environment – both within and without – into consideration. It's not the form of treatment itself that makes it holistic but the underlying awareness behind the treatment that's administered – seeing health or illness as the product of many interrelated forces in our lives.

This suggests that there's a place for all kinds of health care in a holistic context – including standard medical approaches – blood tests, body scans, surgeries and pharmaceutical medications. While it's true that conventional medical approaches are strongly oriented towards measuring and eliminating symptoms, and tend not to see the body in terms of a larger whole, these tools and techniques can still be used in a holistic way. This is something that you, the patient, can bring to it.

> *It's not the form of treatment itself that makes it holistic but the underlying awareness behind the treatment that's administered – seeing health or illness as the product of many interrelated forces in our lives.*

Just as conventional medicine can be part of a holistic health approach, acupuncture, if used improperly, can become non-holistic. Acupuncture taken out of its theoretical context – through medical dry needling, for example – is one example of this. Living your life in a way that continues to exhaust you and cause your back to spasm, then coming for acupuncture to fix it in a crisis, is another. The current scientific research into acupuncture, which holds great potential to elucidate its mechanisms and effects, simultaneously has the potential to strip it of his holistic essence by isolating points and treatments and applying them with a non-holistic understanding.

Ultimately, we are the ones who can choose to make our health – and our treatments – holistic.

## Approaches to Healing

Because physicians are so specialized and so rushed, acupuncturists and other alternative health providers are increasingly becoming the default overseers of people's care. Serving as an advocate, the acupuncturist is often the one helping patients determine which specific medical specialty or combination of approaches they may require. Quite apart from the effectiveness of acupuncture itself, patients are finding in it an environment of trust, inclusion and empowerment that is sorely missing in their experience of conventional medicine. Having this role default to acupuncturists is not the ideal situation.

Many physicians today are caught in a system that they themselves don't like. Doctors wish to spend more time with their patients, but they can't afford to do that. They often send patients for excessive and invasive testing not because it's their choice but because it's required by insurers or to protect themselves legally. Specialization is necessary because the volume of medical knowledge is too vast for a single doctor to hold. Yet this unfortunately exacerbates the tendency to see the body as a collection of unrelated parts.

> *Quite apart from the effectiveness of acupuncture itself, patients are finding in it an environment of trust, inclusion and empowerment that is sorely missing in their experience of conventional medicine.*

Mainstream medicine excels at treating emergencies and severe health crises, including highly advanced pathologies that have gone far beyond the point of healing through less invasive approaches. If you break a bone or require a hip replacement, you want conventional medicine to fix it. For serious, advanced diseases like cancer and impending heart attack, conventional medicine has tools to diagnose and treat you and save your life.

For most of what ails us for most of our lives – fatigue, stress, depression, anxiety, insomnia, acid reflux, pain syndromes, allergies, colds, and aging itself – conventional medicine does not provide the best answer. And to recover from a medical intervention, you also need to seek out complementary therapies – drawing upon acupuncture, massage, herbs, and nutrition, among others – to restore your functional integrity and health.

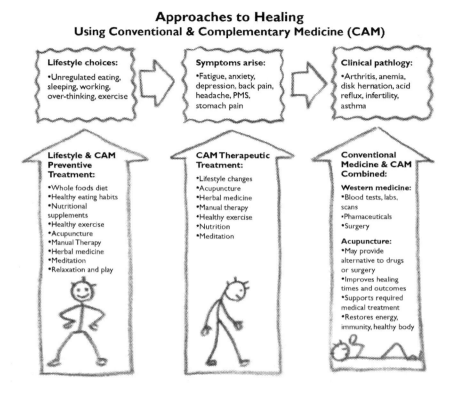

**Approaches to Healing**
**Using Conventional & Complementary Medicine (CAM)**

**Lifestyle choices:**
•Unregulated eating, sleeping, working, over-thinking, exercise

**Symptoms arise:**
•Fatigue, anxiety, depression, back pain, headache, PMS, stomach pain

**Clinical pathlogy:**
•Arthritis, anemia, disk hernation, acid reflux, infertility, asthma

**Lifestyle & CAM Preventive Treatment:**
•Whole foods diet
•Healthy eating habits
•Nutritional supplements
•Healthy exercise
•Acupuncture
•Manual Therapy
•Herbal medicine
•Meditation
•Relaxation and play

**CAM Therapeutic Treatment:**
•Lifestyle changes
•Acupuncture
•Herbal medicine
•Manual therapy
•Healthy exercise
•Nutrition
•Meditation

**Conventional Medicine & CAM Combined:**

**Western medicine:**
•Blood tests, labs, scans
•Phamaceuticals
•Surgery

**Acupuncture:**
•May provide alternative to drugs or surgery
•Improves healing times and outcomes
•Supports required medical treatment
•Restores energy, immunity, healthy body

Acupuncture and other non-conventional health care modalities have been termed "complementary and alternative medicine" (CAM) by the National Institutes of Health.[2] Using them in tandem with conventional medicine is the most effective approach to health care.

Having been disappointed by conventional medicine, some patients reject it completely, seeking only alternative approaches like acupuncture. I'm an acupuncturist but I'm also a patient like everyone else. My personal preference as a patient is to keep myself as healthy as possible through acupuncture, diet, exercise and a balanced lifestyle, and to use a range of treatments when I do become sick or injured.

I've often used acupuncture to help relieve the effects of stress, alleviate insomnia, strengthen my immune system, heal a sprain or muscle strain, and overcome fatigue. But when I've suffered from infections or injuries, I've been grateful for antibiotics and pain relievers and surgical procedures.

We want to keep the tools of modern medicine available to us. As patients we need to learn to combine approaches as needed, working thoughtfully and respectfully in partnership with our doctors and other providers.

If you have something potentially serious, it's essential to consult a Western medical doctor right away. Use medical screening as needed to rule out conditions that require timely medical intervention. Having done that, use acupuncture for treatment before resorting to drugs and surgery that may cause you more problems than they help.

> *As patients we need to learn to combine approaches as needed, working thoughtfully and respectfully in partnership with our doctors and other providers.*

Doctors may request scans or tests to rule out serious problems, but sometimes endless screening is done only because the doctor can't find anything wrong and doesn't know what else to do. Medications are given just to see if they help at times when no diagnosis has been made.

Acupuncture diagnosis identifies patterns of imbalance that are causing symptoms but aren't yet clinically measurable by Western medicine. Pathologies have to be somewhat advanced to be detected using conventional medicine tools. The system of acupuncture is able to understand the problems that haven't yet developed to that level, and to treat them before they become worse.

For most common ailments, start with acupuncture and let it relieve your pain and other symptoms naturally by restoring balance and improving your health.

## Treating the Whole Person

There is more to health than the physical body alone. True health includes body, mind, emotions and, yes, spirit. In the West, we separate these parts and consider illness to be mainly physical. Even mental and emotional problems are frequently treated physically with medications: anti-depressants, mood stabilizers, sleeping pills, painkillers and sedatives of various kinds. While these treatments may at times be helpful and even life-saving, they are primarily symptom-killers that do not get to the root cause of the problem to heal it.

Looking at the whole person provides a very different perspective on illness and allows for truly healing treatment. Patients frequently arrive for acupuncture complaining of whole body pain they can't explain. When you review their history you often find that it traces back to a much earlier injury. Because the original injury never fully healed, the body moves into compensatory structural patterns and creates inflammatory processes that become chronic.

Frequently, the location of pain is not the site of the original injury. To resolve it the treatment must go beyond the symptomatic area. I treated a woman suffering from severe neck and head pain by balancing her tailbone, which had been injured decades earlier in repeated falls while skiing. No amount of therapy to her head or neck on its own had worked to relieve her pain. The tailbone injury was pulling the whole spine and its related soft tissues out of balance all the way up into the neck, the muscular attachments to the skull and around the head.

Another woman had suffered from severe, relentless headaches since having a hysterectomy a few years prior to coming for acupuncture. By treating the scar tissue in her lower abdomen, her headache was immediately and permanently relieved.

Commonly there is unconscious unresolved emotional shock and trauma held in the body at the site of an injury. For the physical pain to heal, the emotional shock must be effectively treated as well. Both physical and emotional symptoms can arise from an earlier loss or trauma. Anxiety, depression, digestive problems – can all have an emotional component from the past or the present.

At times, in response to acupuncture treatment, old symptoms, emotions, or traumatic memories may emerge. This is referred to as a "healing crisis." The body is releasing trapped emotions or old injuries. The symptoms are temporary and through their release, healing takes place. The healing crisis

*Both physical and emotional symptoms can arise from an earlier loss or trauma. Anxiety, depression, digestive problems – can all have an emotional component from the past or the present.*

can be seen when a patient experiences emotions arising in response to treatment – like the sadness I myself felt when I first had acupuncture. Other times a patient may feel anger arising after treatment, or he might go into a dream-like state in which images of old scenes – traumas or injuries from any stage of life – come back to his mind, along with the associated feelings. As a woman's back pain is treated she may find herself sobbing as she relives her childhood experience of being hit by a car. Healing the back pain involves resolving the old emotional trauma as well. To treat any of these conditions effectively, the underlying emotional stress or trauma must also be treated. Acupuncture works on all these levels.

## Change Your Approach to Medicine

Our medical system itself has a life of its own, influenced not only by medical needs but by financial interests as well. Fear is frequently stoked to get patients in for exhaustive, profitable testing or simply to sell stories in the media. I once read about a for-profit business that was rolling RVs into the parking lots of shopping malls and offering free scans to healthy people. Why free? Because the type of scan they were using, a PET (positron emission tomography) scan, will almost always reveal something unusual within the body– most of which is benign and would never have caused a problem. Virtually every patient was being referred for further testing and procedures that were lucrative for the providers. Other business models allow doctors to make a profit on scans to which they refer patients, many of which are unnecessary.

Preventive medicine is not a series of screenings. Living without any consideration for diet, exercise or rest and then getting scanned regularly just to make sure no disease has developed is not a great health plan. This system is unsustainable in any case – as we are seeing more and more. The costs are too high, the benefits too few, and the mistakes all

> *Preventive medicine is not a series of screenings. Living without any consideration for diet, exercise or rest and then getting scanned regularly just to make sure no disease has developed is not a great health plan.*

too common and disastrous. We are staying alive longer but with much lower quality of life, including cognitive decline, physical ailments, painful and costly medical interventions and inhumane end-of-life care.[3] Letting our health go and then falling back on drugs and surgeries does not make us healthier, though it may keep us living longer – but in what condition?

You don't have to wait for the system to change. You can change the system right now simply by changing your approach. This begins with nurturing your health on the "front end" rather than solely chasing illness and disease on the "back end" once it has become a crisis. Then, the doctors won't be so overworked that they don't have time to spend with you. They'll be seeing the patients they really need to see. More doctors will adopt an integrative approach to medicine when you take the lead and show them you want that. Insurers can be persuaded to provide more coverage for complementary treatments when they see how much they can save by helping to keep us healthy. This trend has already begun.

Be aware that there are many financial interests benefitting from our "sickness care" and the opposition to this shift can be strong from these quarters. Likewise, as we increasingly embrace "wellness care," there are other financial interests seeking to sell us treatments and products that we may not need either. The key to healing ourselves – and our medical system – is for us to manage our own health consciously, proactively, thoughtfully and responsibly.

> *The key to healing ourselves – and our medical system – is for us to manage our own health consciously, proactively, thoughtfully and responsibly.*

## Beyond the White Coat: The Empowered Patient

We are outgrowing the old model of doctor-patient relationship. In that approach, the doctor wears the white coat symbolizing his or her authority, and the patient trusts the doctor implicitly, following every instruction that is given.

The doctors and health care providers we consult *are* authorities in their own disciplines, but we are the authorities in our own lives and of our own bodies. Giving over all our own power to doctors is as inappropriate as not recognizing and respecting their knowledge and skills. It's time for doctors (and acupuncturists) to "take off the white coat" and for patients to take the seat of their own authority. As a patient you need to do your due diligence, put together a health care program that works for you, seek out competent providers, think critically about the advice you receive, and then make your own – well-informed – decisions.

One day, I glanced at a television show that was hosted by doctors. A team of guest doctors in white coats were presenting a new "diet." Like many new trends and fad diets, this one had a name and book to go with it. As I watched, the doctors showed slides with kinds of foods to eat and percentages of carbohydrates, fats and proteins you should have your diet. What the diet boiled down to was: "Eat whole, unprocessed, well-prepared foods in balance."

Every day there are new headlines, diets, and fads that sensationalize "discoveries" that amount to scientific validation of things we already knew instinctively, logically and experientially. On the other hand, the health "news" keeps changing. One day we read that coffee is bad for us and try to stop drinking it. The next day we read that coffee has anti-oxidants and is good for us. One report says alcohol is bad and the next says alcohol prevents heart disease and extends life. One year we're running for the trans-fatty acids to avoid cholesterol, a few years later we're running away from those (now proven harmful) trans-fatty acids and recognizing that our body actually needs cholesterol, in balance.

We don't need to wait for science to prove that whole foods are healthy, that sleep is beneficial, and that exercise promotes health. Likewise, we don't need to wait for science to prove how acupuncture works in order to use it for our health. When the results come out, they are validating, but most importantly we can discover for ourselves what "works" and makes us healthier – and follow that.

> *We don't need to wait for science to prove that whole foods are healthy, that sleep is beneficial, and that exercise promotes health. Likewise, we don't need to wait for science to prove how acupuncture works in order to use it for our health.*

Holistic health care, while incorporating both conventional and complementary medicine, takes all levels of ourselves into account – not only the physical body. It emphasizes living in a way that generates and sustains health. It provides you with a range of therapeutic tools to use for restoring health, and give you the ability to choose and assess providers, stage and combine modalities, and to assess and evaluate your progress.

You don't have to be limited by medical prognoses for your pain that tell you that there is no cure for what ails you, and that you just have to "live with it." By learning when and how to use conventional medical screening, pharmaceutical medications, surgeries and other interventions, and when to use acupuncture and other complementary approaches, you can live longer and healthier than you ever imagined possible.

# FREQUENTLY ASKED QUESTIONS

· · · · · · · · · · · · · · · · · · · · ·

**What does acupuncture treat?**

Acupuncture activates the body's innate self-healing abilities. You can use it for almost any condition as well as preventively, to maintain health. The more chronic the condition, the harder it is to heal, and the longer it may take.

## Conditions Commonly Treated with Acupuncture

Pain Syndromes:
- Back and Neck pain
- Rotator cuff injuries
- Frozen shoulder
- Sports Injuries
- Migraines/headaches
- Sciatica
- Fibromyalgia
- Tendonitis: Tennis elbow & Golfer's elbow
- TMJ
- Muscle Cramps
- Restless Legs Syndrome (RLS)
- Arthritis
- Carpal Tunnel Syndrome
- Degenerative Disc Disorders
- TMJ

Upper Respiratory Problems:
- Allergies
- Asthma
- Bronchitis
- Common Cold and Flu
- Sinusitis

Skin Problems:
- Acne
- Dry Skin
- Eczema
- Itching
- Psoriasis
- Rash

Mental/Emotional Disorders:
- Anxiety
- Depression
- Irritability
- Mood Swings
- Panic Attacks

Sleep and Metabolic Disorders:
- Exhaustion and Fatigue
- Insomnia
- Thyroid Dysfunction
- Adrenal Fatigue
- Diabetes Type 2
- Weight Gain

Gastrointestinal Disorders:
- Abdominal Bloating
- Acid Reflux
- Blood sugar imbalance
- Constipation

- Diarrhea
- Excessive hunger
- Hemorrhoids
- Irritable Bowel Syndrome
- Nausea

Reproductive and Urogenital System Disorders:
- Urinary Tract Infection
- Incontinence
- Kidney Stones
- Nighttime Urination
- Urinary Frequency
- Interstitial Cystitis
- Infertility
- Irregular Menstruation
- Menstrual Cramps
- Morning Sickness
- Premenstrual Syndrome (PMS)
- Uterine Fibroids
- Ovarian Cysts
- Polycystic Ovarian Syndrome (PCOS)
- Menopausal Syndrome
- Hot Flashes
- Erectile Dysfunction
- Prostatitis
- Low Sex Drive

Cardiovascular Disorders
- Circulatory Problems
- Heart Disease
- High or Low Blood Pressure

Other Conditions
- General Well-Being
- Immune System Support

- Immune System Support
- Chronic Fatigue
- Smoking Cessation
- Substance Abuse Recovery
- Tinnitus
- Vertigo
- Post-Surgical Recovery

**Is acupuncture safe?**

When performed by a licensed acupuncturist, acupuncture is extremely safe. All needles used are sterile, disposable and used only once. There is virtually no chance of infection occurring as a result of acupuncture treatment. The needles are generally inserted from one eighth to one half inch in depth and retained in position for 20-30 minutes. Needles never touch the organs but work within the superficial layers of skin, fascia and musculature of the body. Blood vessels are flexible and tend to move aside when the fine needles are inserted. In some cases a small blood vessel may be punctured and a bruise may appear for a few days after treatment. Occasionally, patients experience a slight light-headedness immediately after treatment which resolves within minutes.

**Is acupuncture painful?**

Acupuncture needles are extremely thin, and their insertion is virtually painless. In many cases you will not even know that the needles are in place. (Most commonly heard after the initial needle insertion is the phrase, "Is it in?") Once the needles are inserted, they are manipulated gently and at this time there may be a characteristic sensation of tingling, heaviness, or electricity along the meridian. When needles are left in position for 20 minutes or longer (depending on your needs) they are typically not felt at all.

Trigger point release is a special form of needling that involves the stimulation of muscles to relieve painful tension and spasm. It is extremely effective in relieving muscle tension, whether from stress, strain, injury, or surgery. The sensations associated with this type of needling are unique and more pronounced. A trigger point is associated with a tight band within a muscle and it is stimulated to cause the muscle to relax. In the process, the muscle will "twitch" as it's releasing. This is a very unusual sensation and it can be momentarily painful, as you feel a transient "cramp" in the muscle. The muscle may also have a characteristic mild "soreness" for about 24 hours after trigger point release.

The most surprising part of acupuncture for most people is the way they feel during and after treatment. You may fall asleep on the table or enter a state of deep relaxation in which you seem to "float," or "dream." You may have sensations of energy movement throughout the body and along the limbs. Often there are glimpses of inspiration, and creative ideas emerge totally unexpectedly. This experience of an altered, relaxed state is a form of meditative awareness that is characteristic of your natural, centered state of wellness.

**How many treatments will I need?**

The number of treatments required depends on the nature of your complaint. For an acute condition, a single treatment may be sufficient to resolve it. A series of four to ten treatments is effective for many common complaints. Some chronic conditions may require many treatments over time.

Adjunct therapies and self-care techniques can be used to accelerate your progress and reduce the number of treatments required. This may include dietary modifications, nutritional supplementation, herbal medicine, specific exercises, meditation and relaxation techniques, as well as self-massage or home administration of moxibustion.

Unlike conventional Western medical treatment which primarily treats illness after it arises, acupuncture excels in its ability to keep you in balance so that you do not get sick in the first place. By receiving periodic treatments to maintain balance in the body, you can avoid developing serious and debilitating symptoms in the future and sustain greater vitality. Some people receive a monthly treatment to stay in balance. At a minimum, four treatments a year at the change of seasons is very effective in supporting the immune system and keeping you healthy.

## Who can benefit from acupuncture treatment?

Acupuncture is beneficial to people of all ages and all stages of wellness or disease. At every stage of life the human body is able to move towards a state of greater balance and harmony, providing improved health and well-being. People suffering from a wide range of disorders can gain relief from their suffering using acupuncture.

Many people receive acupuncture treatment as a way to ensure that their body will continue to maintain good health and balance. It is not necessary to wait until you have a complaint before receiving acupuncture. One of the great strengths of this approach is its ability to ward off disease by resolving the effects of everyday stress that pulls the body gradually out of balance. A symptom generally arises as a last-stage of a long term accumulation of stresses and imbalances in the body. In acupuncture, elimination of the symptom is just one piece of the overall approach; beyond that it is used to promote and sustain optimal wellness.

## Can children be treated with acupuncture?

Yes. Children are often treated with acupuncture, massage and herbs. Many children are comfortable with acupuncture needles, which are very fine and painlessly inserted. In the treatment of children only a few needles are used. Sometimes the treatment is done using only massage or moxibustion techniques.

Children respond very well to acupuncture and it can help them through the common childhood illnesses in a way that supports their ongoing growth and health. Typical childhood ailments that respond well to acupuncture include colic, pediatric eczema, allergies, colds and flu, bronchitis, asthma, ear infections, bedwetting, restless sleep, hyperactivity, and attention deficit disorders, among others.

## Is acupuncture good for seniors?

Using acupuncture, seniors are able to gain increased vitality and reduction or elimination of unwanted symptoms. Very often senior patients are told there is nothing more that can be done for their condition. Sometimes they experience not being taken seriously by doctors when presenting with physical or mental/emotional conditions that are common at this stage of life, or they are told that it's normal at this age.

Using acupuncture, many of these so-called "normal" conditions can be alleviated. A body at any age can be brought into greater balance, and this is no less true as we grow older. Many common ailments of aging that respond effectively to acupuncture include arthritis, fatigue, back, neck, limb, foot, hand and joint pain, sciatica, anxiety, insomnia, depression, headache, migraine, digestive disorders, low libido, frequency of urination, prostate problems in men, mental fogginess, and sinusitis, among others.

### Can pregnant and lactating women receive acupuncture?

Acupuncture has been used for over 2,000 years to treat pregnant and lactating women. There are a small number acupuncture points that are contraindicated during pregnancy. Acupuncture can help relieve various symptoms occurring during pregnancy, including morning sickness, and provide benefit to the developing fetus. Postpartum mothers are often treated to promote restoration of energy after childbirth, to support healthy lactation, and to balance hormones that commonly lead to postpartum depression and other disorders. Lactating mothers can also take traditional herbal medicine safely when it is prescribed by a qualified herbal medicine practitioner. In fact, small babies are sometimes treated with herbs by supplying those herbs to the mother, who then makes them available to the baby through her breast milk.

### I'm using Western medicine to treat my condition. Can acupuncture interfere with this treatment?

Acupuncture is compatible with most Western medical treatments and will not throw you out of balance or upset the effects of your treatment. If you are on medication, your medication will continue to work. However, your need for certain medications may be reduced as you receive acupuncture, and it's important to stay in touch with your doctor to monitor this. When this happens, it's because you're getting healthier. Acupuncture promotes homeostasis, which is the body's own state of balance. Acupuncture works to balance you; it either helps or is neutral. This is true even for people who are taking psychoactive medications for conditions like depression, anxiety or bipolar disorder. Even patients on anti-coagulant therapy can safely receive acupuncture treatment. While this is the case, there may be specific reasons why your doctor may not want you using acupuncture. If you are in treatment for any serious medical disorder you are advised to consult your physician prior to receiving acupuncture treatment.

## Are there different types of acupuncture?

There are many different styles of acupuncture. Over time, as acupuncture spread throughout Asia, the styles diverged based on different cultures and experiences. All of this knowledge and experience is now becoming available globally. Therefore, different practitioners may utilize very different styles. Any of these approaches will have the capacity to treat your body, mind and spirit, and restore balance.

## What adjunct techniques are used in acupuncture treatment?

### Moxibustion

Moxibustion is the use of a warming herb (mugwort) over selected points along the body's meridian system. There are a number of different methods for applying moxibustion (or "moxa" for short). Indirect moxa involves holding a lighted stick of the herb over the point to warm it. With direct moxa, a salve is applied to the skin to protect it, and a thin thread of loose herb is lit directly over the salve to warm the point. Moxa cones may also be applied to the top of acupuncture needles to provide warmth over the point and through the shaft of the needle. Moxa is used in the treatment of deficiencies, to warm and nourish the body, to relieve local inflammation, and to provide additional energetic stimulation to a point. It is used along with the needles and sometimes on its own.

### Cupping

Cupping involves the application of glass jars that create suction over the skin. A glass jar is held upside down and a flame is inserted and then quickly removed, creating a vacuum that provides suction when applied to the body. (The flame is used only to create the vacuum, and the cups don't feel hot when applied to the skin.) Cupping is used to remove stasis, spasm, pain and congestion in the body. It promotes circulation of blood and lymph in the area where it is applied. It is commonly used to relieve muscular tension as well as for internal disorders, including bronchitis or digestive problems. Cupping may temporarily leave small round red or pink discoloration on the skin, which generally clears within a few days.

### Gua Sha

Gua Sha is a technique that involves rubbing the skin with a smooth surface (typically a ceramic spoon, flat stone or jar lid) in areas where there is congestion or pain. It promotes healthy circulation to the area, relieving pain and tension, and helping to restore proper function to the muscles and the underlying organ systems. It is often used in the case of common cold, head or ear congestion, and neck and muscle pain. Small red dots come to the surface and these typically clear within a few days.

### Electro-Acupuncture

Small electrical currents are sometimes added to the acupuncture needles to create a pronounced effect, particularly for pain relief. The sensation is typically one of "pulsing," where you will feel a painless movement of the muscle near the stimulated needle.

### Tuina Chinese Massage

Tuina techniques may be used to stimulate the body's musculature and circulation. Tuina is a form of massage that releases muscular tension, opens movement in the joints, and promotes circulation.

### Nutrition

Chinese medicine considers nutrition and diet to be an integral part of health and wellness. What we eat, how we eat, and when we eat, as well as what supplements we choose, are considered central to maintaining good health. In Chinese medicine foods have known temperatures and flavors that affect different organ systems. Accordingly, you may be advised by your acupuncturist on what foods to eat and which ones to avoid for your individual condition.

## What do I need to do to prepare for acupuncture treatment?

It's good to make sure you have eaten within 2-4 hours prior to your treatment. Do not come for treatment on an empty stomach. Do not drink alcohol prior to treatment.

## How does acupuncture work for quitting smoking?

If you want to quit smoking, acupuncture can help. It isn't a "magic bullet." You have to want to quit and be motivated. You will be most successful if you use acupuncture in conjunction with a plan. Although smoking is known for its harmful health effects, you are probably using it as a way to relax. In this way, your smoking habit is a kind of self-care. It gives you "permission" to take little breaks from work and time-outs for yourself. The ritual of smoking along with its physiological effects are relaxing for most smokers. If you're going to give it up, it's important to look for other ways to give yourself these breaks and time-outs, and to relax. Ask your family and coworkers to support you so that you take those needed breaks even without smoking as the excuse. Take a short walk outside; have a cup of tea. Start a new exercise that's fun for you; go for massages. Create alternate forms of self-care and relaxation to help you quit smoking.

Along with lifestyle changes, acupuncture can greatly support you as you quit. It does this by reducing physical and emotional cravings for cigarettes, relaxing your nervous system, regulating your blood sugar for stable mood and energy, and restoring your adrenals, frequently depleted due to stress. Acupuncture can also help heal the dryness, heat and damage in the lungs that has come from smoking. You'll breathe better, feel better naturally, and be helped to overcome the addiction. Typically, using acupuncture, it takes just 3-5 days for the addiction itself to clear. After that it's all about supporting your balance so you don't reach for cigarettes habitually to relax and unwind, and repairing smoking-induced damage to the body.

## How does acupuncture work for weight loss?

Acupuncture supports your weight loss in conjunction with healthy dietary choices and exercise. It isn't going to create weight loss if you keep eating junk foods and sitting on the couch – sorry! On the other hand, you may have "tried everything" and done everything right – including diet and exercise – and nothing has worked. Or you may find yourself in a cycle of exhaustion and food cravings that you can't get out of. Acupuncture helps significantly in both of these very common scenarios. When you've done everything right and your weight remains persistently high, your metabolism is out of balance and several different systems are usually not functioning optimally. Often, your adrenals are fatigued and you have high cortisol in the blood, effectively locking fat into the cells and preventing weight loss. Your digestion may be weak and inefficient. When nutrients aren't digested properly they throw off the metabolism and cause weight gain. Your thyroid gland, responsible for metabolic activity, may be weak. Acupuncture restores healthy function in all of these systems, helping them work efficiently and in coordination with one another, as they are meant to do.

When you're in a cycle of stress, exhaustion and food cravings, your adrenals and blood sugar regulation are out of balance. Acupuncture is able to restore strength and healthy function so that food cravings are eliminated and you are able to easily make healthier food choices, sleep more restfully, and find the strength and motivation to exercise.

**What is Chinese herbal medicine and how is it used?**

Chinese herbal formulas are used for a wide range of disorders, from the common cold and flu to allergies, indigestion, morning sickness, insomnia, anxiety, depression and hot flashes. Herbal formulas are often recommended in combination with your acupuncture treatment to increase effectiveness and accelerate progress. They can be taken at home and help to reduce the number of treatments required to resolve a condition. Herbal formulas can be tableted, powdered, or made into liquid tinctures. Decoctions or "teas" are made out of raw herbs at home, and this is an option for those who prefer it.

**What can I expect when I first go for acupuncture?**

Your acupuncturist will typically ask you to complete some forms detailing your main complaints and health history. After having time to review your reason for seeking treatment and your history, and speaking with you, the acupuncturist will feel your pulse on both wrists and look at your tongue. Some acupuncturists will ask you to wear loose-fitting clothes and others will provide you with a treatment robe to change into. Once you're on the treatment table, in addition to pulse and tongue diagnosis, the acupuncturist will often palpate points along the limbs, on the abdomen, or on the back, or wherever you report pain. Having gathered all this information, the acupuncturist selects points and inserts the acupuncture needles. These can be placed anywhere on the body. If you have any fears or concerns about the needles or their placement, you can let the acupuncturist know.

The most used points are those on the lower leg and lower arm, though you may also get points in the torso or even on the face or scalp. They are unlikely to cause any pain. You may be surprised to find yourself becoming very relaxed. Once needles are in place, sometimes moxibustion, a warming herb treatment, will be applied to the points as well. This doesn't hurt and generally induces further relaxation. You will typically get to relax on the table for 20-30 minutes while the needles are retained. This gives your body time to assimilate the effects of the acupuncture treatment. Some acupuncturists, depending on their approach and on your condition, will first treat you facing up, then remove the needles and treat your back as well. If your condition warrants it, you may be treated in a side-lying position or seated in a chair. Complete acupuncture treatment can be administered using points on the front or the back of the body and need not include both.

### What is felt in the pulse?

Acupuncturists use the pulse to understand what is going on inside the body. The rate of the pulse is only one of many qualities that are assessed. By feeling the radial pulse, located on your wrists, the acupuncturist feels three different positions at three different depths. Each position and depth tells a story. For example, a "floating" pulse in the Lung position may indicate upper respiratory problems like infections or allergies. Other qualities may indicate sinus irritation, asthma or bronchitis. If there is phlegm it may be more "slippery." If the entire pulse has a floating quality there may be an acute infection like a cold – which can be detected before you even feel the symptoms yourself. If there is back pain, the last position, corresponding to the Kidneys and the lower back, may be tight or tense. If there is stress, the Liver pulse may be "wiry." If there is stasis of Blood it may be "choppy." The acupuncturist uses the pulse diagnosis as part of the assessment to understand your imbalances and design a treatment plan for you.

**What does my tongue show?**

Most people aren't used to sticking out their tongue and everyone wonders what it is saying. Many people offer spontaneous confessions when asked to show their tongue. ("I just had coffee!") The acupuncturist looks at the tongue for another window into the body. It may be moist or dry. It may be enlarged and swollen, or have teeth marks on the sides, showing fluid retention, a weak Spleen or deficient Kidney yang. It may be thin and dry and red, possibly reflecting Kidney yin deficiency. If the tip of the tongue is red it may indicate heat in the Lungs, relating to bronchitis or asthma, or in the Heart, translating in some cases into anxiety or insomnia. If there is a thick, yellow coating there may be damp heat, or if white and greasy it may indicate dampness and cold. In the patient this would show up as abdominal discomfort, intestinal problems, possible constipation or diarrhea, lack of appetite (or excessive hunger), among other symptoms. If the sides of the tongue are red it may point to heat in the Liver. All of these indicators combine with the pulse and other findings to provide the acupuncturist with a diagnosis and treatment principles upon which to determine point selection for treatment.

**In addition to the pulse and tongue, what other diagnostic methods are used?**

Acupuncturists will listen to the sound of your voice, its strength and tone, and look at any signs on your body including skin tone, hair, markings, posture, movement. They will palpate meridians to feel for tone along their pathways – areas may feel "too tight" or "too soft," suggesting imbalance. Some will feel the abdomen, also known as the "dantian" or "hara," for patterns of muscle tension indicating blockages or deficiencies in certain meridian systems. And they will feel for areas of tension and palpate your areas of pain to understand the patterns and determine a treatment plan for you.

**How can I find a qualified acupuncturist?**

Licensed Acupuncturists in most states use the initials L.Ac. to indicate that they have been properly trained and licensed in their state. Most are also board certified by the National Certification Commission for Acupuncture and Oriental Medicine, and this may be designated as Dipl.

Ac. (NCCAOM), or Dipl. OM (NCCAOM). Chinese herbal medicine diplomacy may also be designated as Dipl. CH (NCCAOM).

The website for the national certifying board provides one of the best databases of acupuncturists nationally (www.nccaom.org). It can be searched by zip code and includes all who are board certified and choose to be listed, and is not a paid or advertising-based list. When you search your zip code you will find a list of Licensed Acupuncturists within your search area with their contact information. I recommend looking at their websites to get a feel for their experience and their style of practice. You can also call and ask if they have experience in treating your condition. For some conditions, such as severe chronic pain, pediatric acupuncture, and women's health issues, including fertility, you may want a more experienced provider. Some acupuncturists focus their practice on a specific condition or age group and it's not uncommon to find acupuncture practices that focus on fertility, women's health, children's health, pain, or sports injuries. However, it's not necessary to locate an acupuncture specialist for most conditions. Unlike Western physicians who frequently specialize, most acupuncturists treat the full range of ages and conditions.

A word of caution: medical doctors, and now even some physical therapists, may also offer acupuncture. In most states they are permitted to do this with little to no training. When offered by doctors it is usually called "Medical Acupuncture" and the physician may use the term Certified Acupuncturist to indicate that a limited training course was attended. Some physicians have taken the initiative to become Licensed Acupuncturists or to otherwise learn the system of acupuncture more thoroughly, and if so they may have greater proficiency. Unless a physician has done so, I suggest going to a Licensed Acupuncturist who has the full training and is acupuncture board certified.

**What is Dry Needling?**

"Dry Needling" is a form of acupuncture. It's the term used for acupuncture when performed in medical settings by doctors or physical therapists to treat musculoskeletal pain. The level of training received by these providers is minimal, and the technique is done outside the context of a complete acupuncture diagnosis and treatment. It is likely to be less effective. I suggest seeing a Licensed Acupuncturist instead.

**Will medical insurance cover acupuncture treatments?**

An increasing number of insurance providers cover acupuncture. Some acupuncturists accept insurance assignment either in-network or out-of-network while others may ask you to submit your own claims for reimbursement. If the acupuncturist accepts assignment, you will only be responsible for a copayment (or coinsurance if out-of-network), plus your deductibles. Some acupuncturists will verify your insurance benefits for you. If not, you can find out yourself by calling your insurance provider directly. Flexible spending accounts for health care usually allow you to use these funds for acupuncture treatment as well.

If you are seeking treatment for injuries sustained in an auto accident, many insurance policies provide reimbursement for acupuncture as well.

**Is low cost acupuncture available?**

If you do not have insurance coverage for acupuncture and if cost is an obstacle for you, low cost acupuncture clinics are increasingly available. Acupuncture colleges have student clinics that provide low cost treatments. Community acupuncture clinics can be located by searching online (search "community acupuncture [your location]". These clinics typically offer acupuncture in group settings for lower cost or a sliding scale fee. Patients relax in reclining chairs or on massage tables while receiving treatment. You may be encouraged to wear or bring shorts and a tee shirt or loose-fitting clothes so that the acupuncture points can be easily reached while you are fully clothed.

**What lifestyle changes are recommended along with acupuncture treatment?**

Based on your individual condition, your acupuncturist will provide you with specific recommendations. Here are a few general guidelines that apply to everyone.

**How and what you eat:**
- Choose whole foods over processed foods.
- Eat regularly. Don't let too many hours pass without eating.
- Eat in peace; breathe and relax. Don't eat on the run or over your computer. Stop and chew your food. If you stay active while

eating, your sympathetic nervous system (fight or flight/stress response) stays active and keeps your digestion from functioning properly. Chewing also adds enzymes to your food, predigesting it and making it easier for your body to assimilate the nutrients.

- Don't skip breakfast. It supplies your body with fuel that you need to begin the day.
- Don't eat too late at night. This leaves your body attempting to digest your food when it's time to rest, which can lead to poor sleep and weight gain.
- Keep in mind that cold and raw foods can weaken the digestion if eaten in excess, as can excessive sugar and cold or iced drinks. Cooked and warm foods are easier to digest. If you need to strengthen your digestion (that includes most people), or if you're suffering from allergies or sinus congestion, focus on warm and cooked foods. Salads and raw vegetables are made more digestible by chewing them well.

**How and when you sleep:**
- Wind down and relax before bed. Don't work right up until bedtime. If you do, you may find it hard to fall or stay asleep, and your sleep may not be as deep and restorative.
- Get enough sleep. Eight hours of sleep at night is recommended.
- Take short naps. If you can lie down for even 10-20 minutes in the afternoon this will restore and reset your body.

**How and when you work:**
- Take regular breaks at work. If you're on the computer all day, stand up and stretch at regular intervals. Lift your eyes from the screen; take some deep breaths.
- Be aware of your posture at work. Even a slight tilt of your head to read something on your desk or to speak on the phone or type or hold a computer mouse can grow into a major pain syndrome over time. Get your ergonomics checked so your work posture keeps you in balance.
- Turn off the work phone and emails when not at work. Yes, it is possible to do this. It's your time and your choice. By doing this

you'll also relieve others of the feeling that they too have to be responsive to calls, texts and emails 24/7.

**How and when you exercise, play and relax:**

- Exercise regularly for fitness. Find an exercise that works for you and do it regularly. If your schedule is really full, see if you can start by walking or biking where you would otherwise drive. Stretch and move in some way every day.
- Give yourself unstructured time. Schedule unscheduled time in your week. You can read, paint, write, meditate, walk in nature, play or relax with friends and family.
- Meditation in some form is essential. Some people prefer "moving meditation" like tai chi. Or you may want to learn to meditate by selecting a class or online resource or app. Even a few minutes of meditation a day goes a long way in keeping you balanced, centered, creative, inspired, healthy and in touch with yourself. Find something that works for you and do it.

# BIBLIOGRAPHY

· · · · · · · · · · · · · · · · · · · · ·

"Acupuncture. NIH Consensus Statement 1997." *The National Institutes of Health (NIH) Consensus Development Program: Acupuncture.* The National Institutes of Health (NIH), 3-5 Nov. 1997.

Audette, Joseph F., and Allison Bailey. *Integrative Pain Medicine: The Science and Practice of Complementary and Alternative Medicine in Pain Management.* Totowa, NJ: Humana, 2008.

*A Barefoot Doctor's Manual: The American Translation of the Official Chinese Paramedical Manual.* Philadelphia: Running, 1977.

Barnes, John F. *Healing Ancient Wounds: The Renegade's Wisdom.* Paoli, PA: Rehabilitation Services, 2000.

Becker, Robert O., and Gary Selden. *The Body Electric: Electromagnetism and the Foundation of Life.* New York: Morrow, 1985.

Betts, Debra. *The Essential Guide to Acupuncture in Pregnancy & Childbirth.* Hove, East Sussex, England: Journal of Chinese Medicine, 2006.

Birch, Stephen. *Shonishin: Japanese Pediatric Acupuncture.* Stuttgart: Thieme, 2011.

Church, Dawson. *The Genie in Your Genes: Epigenetic Medicine and the New Biology of Intention.* Santa Rosa, CA: Elite, 2007.

Connelly, Dianne M. *Traditional Acupuncture: The Law of the Five Elements*. Columbia, MD: Traditional Acupuncture Institute, 1994.

Creel, Herrlee Glessner. *Chinese Thought, from Confucius to Mao Tsê-tung*. Chicago: U of Chicago, 1953.

Deadman, Peter, Mazin Al-Khafaji, and Kevin Baker. *A Manual of Acupuncture*. Hove, East Sussex, England: Journal of Chinese Medicine Publications, 2007.

Dechar, Lorie. *Five Spirits: Alchemical Acupuncture for Psychological and Spiritual Healing*. New York: Chiron Publications/Lantern, 2006.

Denmei, Shudō. *Finding Effective Acupuncture Points*. Seattle: Eastland, 2003.

Elias, Jason, and Katherine Ketcham. *The Five Elements of Self-healing: Using Chinese Medicine for Maximum Immunity, Wellness, and Health*. New York: Harmony, 1998.

Flaws, Bob. *Keeping Your Children Healthy with Chinese Medicine: A Parent's Guide to the Care and Prevention of Common Childhood Diseases*. Boulder, CO: Blue Poppy, 1996.

Flaws, Bob. *The Tao of Healthy Eating: Dietary Wisdom According to Traditional Chinese Medicine*. Boulder, CO: Blue Poppy, 1998.

Grof, Stanislav. *Healing Our Deepest Wounds: The Holotropic Paradigm Shift*. Newcastle, WA: Stream of Experience Productions, 2012.

Guimberteau, Jean-Claude, M.D. "Endoscopy - Microvacuole - Surgeries Videos - Living Matter." *Surgery Videos - Living Matter*. DVD. Endo Vivo Productions.

Guimberteau, Jean-Claude, MD. *Interior Architectures, Exploring the Architecture of the Human Body*. 2012. DVD. Endo Vivo Productions.

Guimberteau, Jean-Claude, MD. *Muscle Attitudes*. 2010. DVD. Endo Vivo Productions.

Guimberteau, Jean-Claude, MD. *Strolling Under The Skin: Images of Living Matter Architecture*. 2005. DVD. ADF Video Productions.

Hammer, Leon, and Karen Bilton. *Handbook of Contemporary Chinese Pulse Diagnosis*. Seattle: Eastland, 2012.

Hicks, Angela, John Hicks, and Peter Mole. *Five Element Constitutional Acupuncture*. Edinburgh: Churchill Livingstone, 2005.

Jarrett, Lonny S. *Nourishing Destiny: The Inner Tradition of Chinese Medicine*. Stockbridge, MA: Spirit Path, 2009.

Kaptchuk, Ted J. *The Web That Has No Weaver: Understanding Chinese Medicine*. New York: Congdon & Weed, 1983.

Kendall, Donald E. *Dao of Chinese Medicine: Understanding an Ancient Healing Art*. Oxford: Oxford UP, 2002.

Keown, Daniel. *The Spark in the Machine: How the Science of Acupuncture Explains the Mysteries of Western Medicine*. Philadelphia: Singing Dragon, 2014.

Kramer, Bruce H., and Cathy Wurzer. *We Know How This Ends: Living While Dying*. University of Minnesota Press, 2015.

Laszlo, Ervin. *Science and the Akashic Field: An Integral Theory of Everything*. Rochester, VT: Inner Traditions, 2004.

Lewis, Randine A. *The Infertility Cure: The Ancient Chinese Wellness Program for Getting Pregnant and Having Healthy Babies*. Boston: Little, Brown, 2004.

Liang, Lifang. *Acupuncture & IVF*. Boulder, CO: Blue Poppy, 2003.

Maciocia, Giovanni. *Diagnosis in Chinese Medicine: A Comprehensive Guide*. Edinburgh: Churchill Livingstone, 2004.

Maciocia, Giovanni. *Obstetrics and Gynecology in Chinese Medicine*. New York: Churchill Livingstone, 1998.

Maciocia, Giovanni. *The Channels of Acupuncture: Clinical Use of the Secondary Channels and Eight Extraordinary Vessels*. Edinburgh: Churchill Livingstone, 2006.

Maciocia, Giovanni. *The Psyche in Chinese Medicine: Treatment of Emotional and Mental Disharmonies with Acupuncture and Chinese Herbs*. Edinburgh: Churchill Livingstone, 2009.

MacPherson, Hugh. *Acupuncture Research: Strategies for Establishing an Evidence Base*. Edinburgh: Churchill Livingstone Elsevier, 2007.

Manaka, Yoshio, Kazuko Itaya, and Stephen Birch. *Chasing the Dragon's Tail: The Theory and Practice of Acupuncture in the Work of Yoshio Manaka*. Brookline, MA: Paradigm Publications, 1995.

Matsumoto, Kiiko, and David Euler. *Kiiko Matsumoto's Clinical Strategies, Vol. 1. in the Spirit of Master Nagano: Vol. 1*. Natick, MA: Kiiko Matsumoto International, 2007.

Northrup, Christiane. *The Wisdom of Menopause: Creating Physical and Emotional Health during the Change*. New York: Bantam, 2012.

Oschman, James L. *Energy Medicine: The Scientific Basis*. Edinburgh: Churchill Livingstone, 2000.

Pischinger, Alfred, and Hartmut Heine. *The Extracellular Matrix and Ground Regulation: Basis for a Holistic Biological Medicine*. Berkeley, CA: North Atlantic, 2007.

Ros, Frank. *The Lost Secrets of Ayurvedic Acupuncture: An Ayurvedic Guide to Acupuncture*. Twin Lakes, WI, U.S.A.: Lotus, 1994.

Schleip, Robert. *Fascia: The Tensional Network of the Human Body: The Science and Clinical Applications in Manual and Movement Therapy.* Edinburgh: Churchill Livingstone/Elsevier, 2012.

Schultz, R. Louis, and Rosemary Feitis. *The Endless Web: Fascial Anatomy and Physical Reality.* Berkeley, CA: North Atlantic, 1996.

Scott, Julian, and Teresa Barlow. *Acupuncture in the Treatment of Children.* Seattle, WA: Eastland, 1999.

Scott, Julian, and Teresa Barlow. *Herbs in the Treatment of Children: Leading a Child to Health.* St. Louis, MO: Churchill Livingstone, 2003.

Seem, Mark. *Acupuncture Physical Medicine: An Acupuncture Touchpoint Approach to the Treatment of Chronic Fatigue, Pain, and Stress Disorders.* Boulder, CO: Blue Poppy, 2000.

Seem, Mark. *A New American Acupuncture: Acupuncture Osteopathy, the Myofascial Release of the Bodymind's Holding Patterns.* Boulder, CO: Blue Poppy, 1993.

Tolle, Eckhart. *The Power Of Now: A Guide to Spiritual Enlightenment.* Novato, CA: New World Library, 1999.

Travell, Janet G., and David G. Simons. *Myofascial Pain and Dysfunction: The Trigger Point Manual.* Baltimore: Williams & Wilkins, 1983.

Travell, Janet G., and David G. Simons. *Myofascial Pain and Dysfunction. the Trigger Point Manual: The Lower Extremities.* Baltimore: Williams & Wilkins, 1992.

Travell, Janet G. *Office Hours: Day and Night; the Autobiography of Janet Travell, M.D.* New York: World Pub., 1968.

Unschuld, Paul U. *Huang Di Nei Jing Su Wen: Nature, Knowledge, Imagery in an Ancient Chinese Medical Text.* Berkeley: U of California, 2003.

Unschuld, Paul U. *Medicine in China: A History of Ideas.* Berkeley: U of California, 1985.

Unschuld, Paul U. *Medicine in China--the Nan-ching: The Classic of Difficult Issues.* Berkeley: U of California, 1986.

Unschuld, Paul U. *What Is Medicine? Western and Eastern Approaches to Healing.* Berkeley, CA: U of California, 2009.

Veith, Ilza. *The Yellow Emperor's Classic of Internal Medicine; Chapters 1-34 Translated from the Chinese with an Introductory Study by Ilza Veith. New Ed.* Berkeley: California UP; London: Cambridge UP, 1966.

West, Zita. *Acupuncture in Pregnancy and Childbirth.* Edinburgh: Churchill Livingstone, 2001.

World Health Organization (WHO). "Acupuncture: Review and Analysis of Reports on Controlled Clinical Trials." Comp. Xiaorui Zhang. (2003): 1-87. 1996. Web.

Zeng, Bai-Yun, Kaicun Zhao, and Fan-rong Liang, eds. *Neurobiology of Acupuncture.* Vol. III. Oxford: Elsevier, 2013.

# ENDNOTES

· · · · · · · · · · · · · · · · · · · ·

## Chapter 1

[1] Zhao, ZQ. "Neural Mechanism Underlying Acupuncture Analgesia." *Progress in Neurobiology* 85.4 (2008): 355-75.

[2] Zhang, W.T., Z. Jin, F. Luo, L. Zhang, Y.W. Zeng, and J.S. Han. "Evidence from Brain Imaging with FMRI Supporting Functional Specificity of Acupoints in Humans." *Neurosci Lett* 354.1 (2004): 50-53.

[3] Flachskampf, F.A., J. Gallasch, O. Gefeller, J. Gan, J. Mao, et. al. "Randomized Trial of Acupuncture to Lower Blood Pressure." *Circulation* 115.24 (2007): 3121-129.

[4] For example, Hammer, L. "Phlegm Misting-Disturbing the Orifices and Mitral Valve Prolapse." *European Journal of Oriental Medicine* 7.3 (2013): 1-6. *Dragon Rises*. EJOM, 2013.

[5] Unschuld, Paul U. *Medicine in China: A History of Ideas*. Berkeley: University of California, 1985, pp. 78-79.

## Chapter 2

[1] Saini, A. "Epigenetics: Genes, Environment and the Generation Game." *The Guardian*. 6 Sept. 2014; "Neuroplasticity: An Extraordinary Discovery of the Twentieth Century." *Neuroplasticity: An Extraordinary Discovery of the Twentieth Century*. Web. 22 Feb. 2015. http://www.learninginfo.org/neuroplasticity.htm

[2] Unschuld, Paul U. *Medicine in China: A History of Ideas*. Berkeley: U of California, 1985, p. 72

[3] See Chapter Four: Acupuncture: An Ancient Healing Technique, for more on the development of TCM in 20th century China.

[4] Gori, Luigi, and Fabio Firenzuoli. "Ear Acupuncture in European Traditional Medicine." *Evid Based Complement Alternat Med*. 4.(Suppl 1) (2007): 13-16.

5    Oleson, T.D., R.J. Kroening, and D.E. Bresler. "An Experimental Evaluation of Auricular Diagnosis: The Somatotopic Mapping of Musculoskeletal Pain at Ear Acupuncture Points." *Pain* 8.2 (1980): 217-29.

6    Richards, D., and J. Marley. "Stimulation of Auricular Acupuncture Points in Weight Loss." *Aust Fam Physician* 27.Suppl 2 (1998): S73-77; Kang, O. S., G. H. Johng, H. Kim, J. W. Kim, et. al. "Neural Substrates of Acupuncture in the Modulation of Cravings Induced by Smoking-related Visual Cues: An FMRI Study." *Psychopharmacology (Berl.)* 228.1 (2013): 119-27.

7    Plunkett, A., A. Turabi, and I. Wilkinson. "Battlefield Analgesia: A Brief Review of Current Trends and Concepts in the Treatment of Pain in US Military Casualties from the Conflicts in Iraq and Afghanistan." *Pain Manag.* May; 2.3 (2012): 231-38; Elwy, A. R., J. M. Johnston, and Et Al. "A Systematic Scoping Review of Complementary and Alternative Medicine Mind and Body Practices to Improve the Health of Veterans and Military Personnel." *Med Care* 52(12 Suppl 5) (2014): S70-82; Chang, B. H., and E. Sommers. "Acupuncture and Relaxation Response for Craving and Anxiety Reduction among Military Veterans in Recovery from Substance Use Disorder." *Am J Addict.* 23.2 (2014): 129-36.

8    Travell, Janet G., and David G. Simons. *Myofascial Pain and Dysfunction: The Trigger Point Manual.* Baltimore: Williams & Wilkins, 1983. p. 951

9    Travell, Janet G. *Office Hours: Day and Night; the Autobiography of Janet Travell, M.D.* New York: World Pub., 1968. p. 257

10   Audette, Joseph F., and Allison Bailey. *Integrative Pain Medicine: The Science and Practice of Complementary and Alternative Medicine in Pain Management.* Totowa, NJ: Humana, 2008. p.116

11   Seem, Mark. *Acupuncture Physical Medicine: An Acupuncture Touchpoint Approach to the Treatment of Chronic Fatigue, Pain, and Stress Disorders.* Boulder, CO: Blue Poppy, 2000.

12   Gobbo, M., N.A. Maffiuletti, C. Orizio, and M.A. Minetto. "Muscle Motor Point Identification Is Essential for Optimizing Neuromuscular Electrical Stimulation Use." *J Neuroeng Rehabil* 11.17 (2014): 11-17.

13   Liu, Y., M. Varela, and R. Oswald. "The Correspondence between Some Motor Points and Acupuncture Loci." *Am J Chin Med* 3.4 (1975): 347-58.

## Chapter 3

1    Meridian abbreviations used:
     LU: Lung
     LI: Large Intestine
     K: Kidney
     BL: Urinary Bladder
     LV: Liver

GB: Gallbladder

HT: Heart

SI: Small Intestine

PC: Pericardium

TH: Triple Heater

SP: Spleen

ST: Stomach

CV: Conception Vessel (Ren)

GV: Governing Vessel (Du)

2    Based on clinical experience and suggestive research data. Conclusive scientific proof is not yet available. For some representative scientific reports see: Cui, W., J. Li, W. Sun, and J. Wen. "Effect of Electroacupuncture on Oocyte Quality and Pregnancy for Patients with PCOS Undergoing in Vitro Fertilization and Embryo Transfer vitro Fertilization and Embryo Transfer." *Zhongguo Zhen Jiu* 31.8 (2011): 687-91; Huang, D. M., and Et Al. "Acupuncture for Infertility: Is It an Effective Therapy?" *Chin J Integr Med* 17.5 (2011): 386-95; Anderson, B., and L. Rosenthal. "Acupuncture and in Vitro Fertilization: Critique of the Evidence and Application to Clinical Practice." *Complement Ther Clin Pract* 19 (2013): 1-5; Hu, M., Y. Zhang, H. Ma, and Et Al. "Eastern Medicine Approaches to Male Infertility." *Semin Reprod Med* 41.4 (2013): 301-10.

## Chapter 4

1    The shorthand term "Neijing" is commonly used for this text. It's complete title is: Huang Di Nei Jing Su Wen. The Ma-wang-tui graves, discovered in China in the 1970s, provide unedited texts along with artifacts dating to 168 B.C.

2    Unschuld, Paul U. *Huang Di Nei Jing Su Wen: Nature, Knowledge, Imagery in an Ancient Chinese Medical Text.* Berkeley: U of California, 2003, pp. 1-3.

3    In its current form the *Neijing* is comprised of two parts, the *Su Wen* (Simple Questions) and the *Ling Shu* (Spiritual Pivot), each 81 chapters long.

4    The Nanjing, "The Classic of Difficult Issues," was compiled in the first century CE, possibly in an effort to resolve the numerous contradictions in the Neijing. The Nanjing is another important early treatise on the practice of acupuncture, upon which many subsequent commentaries are based.

5    Unschuld, Paul U. *Medicine in China: A History of Ideas.* Berkeley: U of California, 1985, p. 45, p. 97; Unschuld, Paul U. *What Is Medicine? Western and Eastern Approaches to Healing.* Berkeley, CA: U of California, 2009, p. 46

6    See Chapter Two: How Acupuncture Heals, for more information about acupuncture styles.

7    Ros, Frank. *The Lost Secrets of Ayurvedic Acupuncture: An Ayurvedic Guide to Acupuncture.* Twin Lakes, WI, U.S.A.: Lotus, 1994; Gori, L., and F. Firenzouli.

"Ear Acupuncture in European Traditional Medicine." *Evidence-Based Compl Altern Med* 4.S1 (2007): 13-16. *Ear Acupuncture in European Traditional Medicine.*

[8]  Reston, James. "Now, About My Operation in Peking." *New York Times* (1971): 1-2.

[9]  "Acupuncture. NIH Consensus Statement 1997." *The National Institutes of Health (NIH) Consensus Development Program: Acupuncture.* The National Institutes of Health (NIH), 3-5 Nov. 1997.

[10]  World Health Organization (WHO). "Acupuncture: Review and Analysis of Reports on Controlled Clinical Trials." Comp. Xiaorui Zhang. (2003): 1-87. 1996.

[11]  Duran, Brenda. "Acupuncture Today in China: Part I." *Acupuncture Today* 14.1 (2013): 1. Jan. 2013.

[12]  Reddy, Sumathi. "A Top Hospital Opens Up to Chinese Herbs as Medicines." *The Wall Street Journal.* Dow Jones & Company, 21 Apr. 2014.

[13]  Chernyak, G.V., and D.I. Sessler. "Perioperative Acupuncture and Related Techniques." *Anesthesiology* 102.5 (2005): 1031-078.

[14]  Zhou, J., H. Chi, T.O. Cheng, T.Y. Chen, Y.Y. Wu, W.X. Zhou, W.D. Shen, and L. Yuan. "Acupuncture Anesthesia for Open Heart Surgery in Contemporary China." *Int J Cardiol* 12-6 150.1 (2011); Unschuld, Paul U. *Medicine in China: A History of Ideas.* Berkeley: U of California, 1985, pp. 360-366

## Chapter 5

[1]  Bhasin, Manoj K., Jeffery A. Dusek, Bei-Hung Chang, Marie G. Joseph, John W. Denninger, Gregory L. Fricchione, Herbert Benson, and Towia A. Libermann. "Relaxation Response Induces Temporal Transcriptome Changes in Energy Metabolism, Insulin Secretion and Inflammatory Pathways." PLOS ONE. doi: 10.1371/journal.pone.0062817 (2013).

[2]  There are many studies that show this. Here is one illustrative example: Brinkhaus, B., C. M. Witt, S. Jena, K. Linde, et al. "Acupuncture in Patients with Chronic Low Back Pain: A Randomized Controlled Trial." *Arch Intern Med* 166.4 (2006): 450-57.

[3]  Paterson, C., and P. Dieppe. "Characteristic and Incidental (placebo) Effects in Complex Interventions Such as Acupuncture." *BMJ* 330.7501 (2005): 1202-205.

[4]  Manyanga, T., M. Froese, R. Zarychanski, A. Abou-Setta, et. al. "Pain Management with Acupuncture in Osteoarthritis: A Systematic Review and Meta-analysis." *BMC Complement Altern Med* 14 (1): 312 (2014); Manheimer, E., K. Linde, L. Lao, L. Bouter, and B. Berman. "Meta-analysis: Acupuncture for Osteoarthritis of the Knee." *Annals of Internal Medicine* 146.12 (2007)

5    Research Group of Acupuncture Anesthesia PMC. "The Role of Some Neurotransmitters of the Brain in Finger-Acupuncture Analgesia." *Scientia Sinica* 17 (1974): 112-30.

6    For example, Elder, C., C. Ritenbaugh, M. Aickin, et al. "Reductions in Pain Medication Use Associated with Traditional Chinese Medicine for Chronic Pain." *Permanente Journal* 16.3 (2012): 18-23.

7    Lin, J.G., and W.L. Chen. "Acupuncture Analgesia: A Review of Its Mechanisms of Actions." *Am J Chin Med* 36.4 (2008): 635-45., Han, J.S. "Acupuncture: Neuropeptide Release Produced by Electrical Stimulation of Different Frequencies." *Trends in Neurosciences* 26.1 (2003): 17-22; Chen, X.H., and J.S. Han. "Analgesia Induced by Electroacupuncture of Different Frequencies Is Mediated by Different Types of Opioid Receptors. Another Cross-tolerance Study." *Behavioural Brain Research* 47.2 (1992): 143-49.

8    Zhao, ZQ. "Neural Mechanism Underlying Acupuncture Analgesia." *Progress in Neurobiology* 85.4 (2008): 355-75.

9    Zhang, W.T., Z. Jin, F. Luo, L. Zhang, Y.W. Zeng, and J.S. Han. "Evidence from Brain Imaging with FMRI Supporting Functional Specificity of Acupoints in Humans." *Neurosci Lett* 354.1 (2004): 50-53.; Napadow, V., N. Makris, J. Liu, N.W. Kettner, K.K. Kwong, and K.K. Hui. "Effects of Electroacupuncture versus Manual Acupuncture on the Human Brain as Measured by FMRI." *Human Brain Mapping* 24.3 (2005): 193-205.

10    Zhang, R.X., L. Lao, X. Wang, A. Fan, L. Wang, K. Ren, and B.M. Berman. "Electroacupuncture Attenuates Inflammation in a Rat Model." *J Altern Complement Med* 11.1 (2005): 135-42.

11    Kim, H.W., D.K. Uh, S.Y. Yoon, D.H. Roh, Y.B. Kown, H.J. Han, et. al. "Low-frequency Electroacupuncture Suppresses Carrageenan-induced Paw Inflammation in Mice via Sympathetic Post-ganglionic Neurons, While High-frequency EA Suppression Is Mediated by the Sympathoadrenal Medullary Axis." *Brain Res Bill* 75.5 (2008): 698-705.

12    Pomeranz, B., and D. Chiu. "Naloxone Blockade of Acupuncture Analgesia: Endorphin Implicated." *Life Sci* 19.11 (1976): 1757-762; Langevin, H.M., D.L. Churchill, J. Wu, G.J. Badger, J.A. Yandow, J.R. Fox, and M.H. Krag. "Evidence of Connective Tissue Involvement in Acupuncture." *Faseb J.* 16 (2002): 872-74.

13    Inoue, M., H. Kitakoji, T. Yano, N. Ishizaki, et. al. "Acupuncture Treatment for Low Back Pain and Lower Limb Symptoms—The Relation between Acupuncture or Electroacupuncture Stimulation and Sciatic Nerve Blood Flow." *Evidence-Based Complementary and Alternative Medicine* 5.2 (2008): 133-43.

14    Napadow, V., N. Kettner, J. Liu, M. Li, K.K. Kwong, M. Vangel, N. Makris, et. al. "Hypothalamus and Amygdala Response to Acupuncture Stimuli in Carpal Tunnel Syndrome." *Pain* 130.3 (2007): 254-66.

15  Cha, M.H., J.S. Choi, S.J. Bai, I. Shim., et. al. "Antiallodynic Effects of Acupuncture in Neuropathic Rats." *Yonsei Med J* 47.3 (2006): 359-66

16  Zeng, Bai-Yun, Kaicun Zhao, and Fan-rong Liang. *Neurobiology of Acupuncture.* Vol. III. Oxford: Elsevier, 2013, pp.134-135

17  Harvard Health Publications. "What Causes Depression?" *Harvard Health Publications Understanding Depression.* Web. 14 Nov 2014

18  Feighner, J.P. "Mechanism of Action of Antidepressant Medication." *Journal of Clinical Psychiatry* 60.4 (1999): 4-13.

19  Sun, H., Y. Zhang, and C.H. Han. "Effects of Electro-acupuncture on the Number and Binding Activity of 5-HT1 and 5-HT2 Receptors in the Cerebral Cortex of Chronic Stress Depression Model Rats." *International Journal of Clinical Acupuncture* 14.2 (2005): 113-18.

20  Schnyer, R.N. "Commentary on the Cochrane Review of Acupuncture for Depression." *EXPLORE: The Journal of Science and Healing* 7.3 (2011): 193-97.

21  Duan, D-M, Y. Tu, S. Jiao, and W. Qin. "The Relevance between Symptoms and Magnetic Resonance Imaging Analysis of the Hippocampus of Depressed Patients given Electro-acupuncture Combined with Fluoxetine Intervention — A Randomized, Controlled Trial." *Chin J Integr Med* 17.3 (2011): 190-99.

22  Zhang, J., J. Chen, J. Chen, X. Li, et. al. "Early Filiform Needle Acupuncture for Poststroke Depression: A Meta-analysis of 17 Randomized Controlled Clinical Trials." *Neural Regen Res* 9.7 (2014): 773-84.

23  Sheline, Y.I., M. Sanghavi, M.A. Mintun, and M.H. Gado. "Depression Duration But Not Age Predicts Hippocampal Volume Loss in Medically Healthy Women with Recurrent Major Depression." *The Journal of Neuroscience* 19.12 (1999): 5034-043.

24  Zeng, Bai-Yun, Kaicun Zhao, and Fan-rong Liang. *Neurobiology of Acupuncture.* Vol. III. Oxford: Elsevier, 2013 p. 206

25  Sun, H., Y. Zhang, and C.H. Han. "Effects of Electro-acupuncture on the Number and Binding Activity of 5-HT1 and 5-HT2 Receptors in the Cerebral Cortex of Chronic Stress Depression Model Rats." *International Journal of Clinical Acupuncture* 14.2 (2005): 113-18.

26  Dos Santos, J.G., Jr., F. Kawagano, M.M. Nishida, et al. "Antidepressive-like Effects of Electroacupuncture in Rats." *Physiology & Behavior* 93.1-2 (2008): 155-59.

27  Vazquez, R., L. Gonzalez-Macias, C. Berlanga, and F.J. Aedo. "Effect of Acupuncture Treatment on Depression: Correlation between Psychological Outcomes and Salivary Cortisol Levels." *Salud Mental* 34 (2011): 21-26.

28  Sun, H., H. Zhao, C. Ma, F. Bao, J. Zhang, et. al. "Effects of Electroacupuncture on Depression and the Production of Glial Cell Line–Derived Neurotrophic Factor Compared with Fluoxetine: A Randomized Controlled Pilot Study." *The Journal of Alternative and Complementary Medicine* 19.9 (2013): 733-39.

29     Eshkevari, L., E. Permaul, and S. E. Mulroney. "Acupuncture Blocks Cold Stress-induced Increases in the Hypothalamus-pituitary-adrenal Axis in the Rat." *Journal of Endocrinology* 17.1 (2013): 95-104, Kim, H., H.J. Park, S.M. Han, D.H. Hahm, H.J Lee, et. al. "The Effects of Acupuncture Stimulation at PC6 (Neiguan) on Chronic Mild Stress-induced Biochemical and Behavioral Responses." *Neuroscience Letters* 460.1 (2009): 56-60, Park, H.J, Y. Chae, J. Jang, I. Shim, H. Lee, and S. Lim. "The Effect of Acupuncture on Anxiety and Neuropeptide Y Expression in the Basolateral Amygdala of Maternally Separated Rats." *Neuroscience Letters* 377.3 (2005): 179-84, Park, H.J, H.J Park, Y. Chae, J.W Kim, H. Lee, and J.H. Chung. "Effect of Acupuncture on Hypothalamic– Pituitary–Adrenal System in Maternal Separation Rats." *Cellular and Molecular Neurobiology* 31.8 (2011): 1123-127.

30     Arranz, L., L. Siboni, and M. De La Fuente. "Improvement of Interleukin 2 and Tumor Necrosis Factor Alpha Release by Blood Leukocytes as Ell as of Plasma Cortisol and Antioxidant Levels after Acupuncture Treatment in Women Suffering Anxiety." *J Appl Biomed* 4.3 (2006): 115-22.

31     Fang, J., Z. Jin, Y. Wang, K. Li, J. Kong, E.E. Nixon, et al. "The Salient Characteristics of the Central Effects of Acupuncture Needling: Limbic-paralimbic-neocortical Network Modulation." *Hum Brain Mapp* 30.4 (2009): 1196-206.

32     Chang, B.H., and E. Sommers. "Acupuncture and Relaxation Response for Craving and Anxiety Reduction among Military Veterans in Recovery from Substance Use Disorder." *Am J Addict* 23.2 (2014): 129-36; Chan, Y.Y., W.Y. Lo, T.C. Li, S.N. Yang, et al. "Clinical Efficacy of Acupuncture as an Adjunct to Methadone Treatment Services for Heroin Addicts: A Randomized Controlled Trial." *Am J Chin Med* 42.3 (2014): 569-86.

33     Bergdahl, L., A. H. Berman, and K. Haglund. "Patients' Experience of Auricular Acupuncture during Protracted Withdrawal." *J Psychiatr Meant Health Nurs* 21.2 (2014): 163-69.

34     CDC. "Insufficient Sleep Is a Public Health Epidemic." *Centers for Disease Control and Prevention*, 13 Jan. 2014; Colten, Harvey R., and Bruce M. Altevogt, eds. "Sleep Disorders and Sleep Deprivation, An Unmet Public Health Problem." *National Academies Press (US)* (2006)

35     Chan, Amanda L. "The Disturbing Side Effect Of Ambien, The No. 1 Prescription Sleep Aid." *The Huffington Post*, TheHuffingtonPost.com,15 Jan. 2014; Liao, J.. "Ambien: The Good, the Bad, the Reality." *The Atlantic*. Atlantic Media Company, 18 June 2013.

36     Zhao, K. "Acupuncture for the Treatment of Insomnia." *Int Rev Neurobiol* 111 (2013): 217-34.

37     Spence, D.W., L. Kayumov, A. Chen, A. Lowe, et. al. "Acupuncture Increases Nocturnal Melatonin Secretion and Reduces Insomnia and Anxiety: A

Preliminary Report." *J Neuropsychiatry Clin Neurosci* 16.1 (2004): 19-28; Han, J.S. "Electroacupuncture: An Alternative to Antidepressants for Treating Affective Diseases?" *Int J Neurosci* 29.1-2 (1986): 79-92; Lee, B. H., J. Y. Ku, R. J. Zaho, H. Y. Kim, C. H. Yang, et al. "Acupuncture at HT7 Suppresses Morphine Self-administration at High Dose through GABA System." *Neurosci Lett* 576 (2014): 34-39.

38  Kung, Y.Y., C.C. Yang, J.H. Chiu, and T.B. Kuo. "The Relationship of Subjective Sleep Quality and Cardiac Autonomic Nervous System in Postmenopausal Women with Insomnia under Auricular Acupressure." *Menopause* 18.6 (2011): 638-45.

39  Lee, S.Y., Y.H. Baek, S.U. Park, et. al. "Intradermal Acupuncture on Shen-men and Nei-kuan Acupoints Improves Insomnia in Stroke Patients by Reducing the Sympathetic Nervous Activity: A Randomized Clinical Trial." *Am J Chin Med* 37.6 (2009): 1013-021.

40  Cabrini, L., L. Gioia, M. Gemma, and Et. Al. "Bispectral Index Evaluation of the Sedative Effect of Acupuncture in Healthy Volunteers." *J Clin Monit Comput* 20.5 (2006): 311-15. 19 Sept. 2006.

41  Winkelman, J.W., O.M. Buxton, J.E. Jensen, et. al. "Reduced Brain GABA in Primary Insomnia: Preliminary Data from 4T Proton Magnetic Resonance Spectroscopy (1H-MRS)." *Sleep* 31.11 (2008): 1499-506.

42  Mitchell, H.A., and D. Weinshenker. "Good Night and Good Luck: Norepinephrine in Sleep Pharmacology." *Biochem Pharmacol* 79.6 (2010): 801-09.

43  Zhou, Y. L., X. Y. Gao, P. Y. Wang, and S. Ren. "Effect of Acupuncture at Different Acupoints on Expression of Hypothalamic GABA and GABA(A) Receptor Proteins in Insomnia Rats." *Zhen Ci Yan Jiu* 37.4 (2012): 302-07.

44  Gooneratne, Nalaka S. "Complementary and Alternative Medicine for Sleep Disturbances in Older Adults." *Clin Geriatr Med* 24.1 (2008): 121-viii. 1 Feb. 2009.

45  Ferracioli-Oda, E., A. Qawasmi, and M.H. Bloch. "Meta-Analysis: Melatonin for the Treatment of Primary Sleep Disorders." *PLOS ONE:* 17 May 2013.

46  Spence, D. W., L. Kayumov, A. Chen, A. Lowe, U. Jain, and Et Al. "Acupuncture Increases Nocturnal Melatonin Secretion and Reduces Insomnia and Anxiety: A Preliminary Report." *The Journal of Neuropsychiatry & Clinical Neurosciences* 16.1 (2004): 19-28.

47  Park, H.J, H.J Park, Y. Chae, J.W Kim, H. Lee, and J.H. Chung. "Effect of Acupuncture on Hypothalamic–Pituitary–Adrenal System in Maternal Separation Rats." *Cellular and Molecular Neurobiology* 31.8 (2011): 1123-127.

48  CDC. "High Blood Pressure Facts." Centers for Disease Control and Prevention, 29 Oct. 2014.

49 Cevik, C., and S. O. Iseri. "The Effect of Acupuncture on High Blood Pressure of Patients Using Antihypertensive Drugs." *Acupunct Electrother Res* 38.1-2 (2013): 1-15.

50 Flachskampf, F.A., J. Gallasch, O. Gefeller, J. Gan, J. Mao, et. al. "Randomized Trial of Acupuncture to Lower Blood Pressure." *Circulation* 115.24 (2007): 3121-129; Crisostomo, M.M., P. Li, S.C. Tjen-A-Looi, and J.C. Longhurst. "Nociceptin in RVLM Mediates Electroacupuncture Inhibition of Cardiovascular Reflex Excitatory Response in Rats." *J Appl Physiol* 98.6 (2005): 2056-063.

51 Tjen-A-Looi, S.C., P. Li, and J.C. Longhurst. "Medullary Substrate and Differential Cardiovascular Responses during Stimulation of Specific Acupoints." *Am J Physiol Regul Integr Comp Physiol* 287.4 (2004): 852-62.

52 Li, P., O. Ayannusi, C. Reid, and J.C. Longhurst. "Inhibitory Effect of Electroacupuncture (EA) on the Pressor Response Induced by Exercise Stress." *Clin Auton Res* 14.3 (2004): 182-88; Tjen-A-Looi, S.C., Z.L. Guo, and J.C. Longhurst. "Medullary GABAergic Mechanisms Contribute to Electroacupuncture Modulation of Cardiovascular Depressor Responses during Gastric Distention in Rats." *Am J Physiol Regul Integr Comp Physiol* 304.5 (2013): 321-32.

53 Li, P., K.F. Pitsillides, S.V. Rendig, H.L. Pan, and J.C. Longhurst. "Reversal of Reflex-induced Myocardial Ischemia by Median Nerve Stimulation: A Feline Model of Electroacupuncture." *Circulation* 97.12 (1998): 1186-194.

54 Hsiao, A-F, S. Tjen-A-Looi, W. Zhou, P. Li, R. Cabatbat, and J.C. Longhurst. "Neural Pathways of Cardiovascular Depressor Reflex during Gastric Distension and Its Modulation by Electroacupuncture." *FASEB J.* 22 (1) (2008): 737.23; Tjen-A-Looi, S.C., P. Li, and J.C. Longhurst. "Role of Medullary GABA, Opioids, and Nociceptin in Prolonged Inhibition of Cardiovascular Sympathoexcitatory Reflexes during Electroacupuncture in Cats." *Am J Physiol Heart Circ Physiol* 293.6 (2007): H3627-3635.

55 Shah, N.D., D.K. Chitkara, R. Locke, et al. "Ambulatory Care for Constipation in the United States, 1993-2004." *Am Jour Gastroent* 103.7 (2008): 1746-753.

56 Iwa, M. "Electroacupuncture at ST-36 Accelerates Colonic Motility and Transit in Freely Moving Conscious Rats." *AJP: Gastrointestinal and Liver Physiology* 290.2 (2006): G285-292.

57 Li, Y. Q., B. Zhu, P.J. Rong, H. Ben, and Y.H. Li. "Neural Mechanism of Acupuncture-modulated Gastric Motility." *World J Gastroenterol* 13.5 (2007): 709-16; Iwa, M., M. Tateiwa, M. Sakita, M. Fujimiya, and T. Takahashi. "Anatomical Evidence of Regional Specific Effects of Acupuncture on Gastric Motor Function in Rats." *Auton Neurosci* 137.1-2 (2007): 67-76.

58 Yu, Z., YB Xia, J. Lin, WJ Yu, and B. Xu. "Influence of Electroacupuncture Stimulation of "tianshu" (ST 25), "quchi" (LI 11) and "shangjuxu" (ST 37) and Their Pairs on Gastric Motility in the Rat." *Zhen Ci Yan Jiu* 38.1 (2013): 40-47.

59    Li, H., L. X. Pei, and J.L. Zhou. "Comparative Observation on Therapeutic Effects between Acupuncture and Western Medication for Diarrhea-predominant Irritable Bowel Syndrome." *Zhongguo Zhen Jiu* 32.8 (2012): 679-82.

60    MacPherson, H., H. Tilbrook, J.M. Bland, K. Bloor, S. Brabyn, et. al. "Acupuncture for Irritable Bowel Syndrome: Primary Care Based Pragmatic Randomised Controlled Trial." *BMC Gastroenterol* 24.12 (2012): 150-67.

61    Chu, W.C., J.C. Wu, D.T. Yew, L. Zhang, et. al. "Does Acupuncture Therapy Alter Activation of Neural Pathway for Pain Perception in Irritable Bowel Syndrome?: A Comparative Study of True and Sham Acupuncture Using Functional Magnetic Resonance Imaging." *J Neurogastroenterol Motil* 18.3 (2012): 305-16.

62    Liu, M.R., R.F. Xiao, Z.P. Peng, et. al. "Effect of Acupuncture at "Zusanli" (ST 36 and "Taichong" (LR 3) on Gastrointestinal Hormone Levels in Rats with Diarrhea Type Irritable Bowel Syndrome." *Zhen Ci Yan Jiu* 37.5 (2012): 363-68.

63    Dundee, J.W., R.G. Ghaly, K.T. Fitzpatrick, G.A. Lunch, and W.P. Abram. "Acupuncture to Prevent Cisplatin-associated Vomiting." *Lancet* 1.1083 (1987); Dundee, J.W., R.G. Ghaly, K.M. Bill, W.N. Chestnut, K.T. Fitzpatrick, and A.G. Lynas. "Effect of Stimulation of the P6 Antiemetic Point on Postoperative Nausea and Vomiting." *Br J Anaesth* 63.5 (1989): 612-18.

64    Lin, X., J. Liang, J. Ren, F. Mu, M. Zhang, and J.D. Chen. "Electrical Stimulation of Acupuncture Points Enhances Gastric Myoelectrical Activity in Humans." *Am J Gastroenterol* 92.9 (1997): 1527-530.

65    Tatewaki, M., C. Strickland, H. Fukada, D. Tsuchida, E. Hoshino, and T. N. Pappas. "Effects of Acupuncture on Vasopressin-induced Emesis in Conscious Dogs." *AJP: Regulatory, Integrative and Comparative Physiology* 288.2 (2005): R401-408; Hu, S., R.M. Stern, and K.L. Koch. "Electrical Acustimulation Relieves Vection-induced Motion Sickness." *Gastroenterology* 102.6 (1992): 1854-858.

66    West, Zita. *Acupuncture in Pregnancy and Childbirth*. Edinburgh: Churchill Livingstone, 2001; Betts, Debra. *The Essential Guide to Acupuncture in Pregnancy & Childbirth*. Hove, East Sussex, England: Journal of Chinese Medicine, 2006

67    Van Den Berg, I., G.C. Kaandorp, J.L. Bosch, et. al. "Cost-effectiveness of Breech Version by Acupuncture-type Interventions on BL 67, including Moxibustion, for Women with a Breech Foetus at 33 Weeks Gestation: A Modelling Approach." *Complement There Med* 18.2 (2010): 67-77; Li, Xun, Jun Hu, Xiaoyi Wang, Huirui Zhang, and Jianping Liu. "Moxibustion and Other Acupuncture Point Stimulation Methods to Treat Breech Presentation: A Systematic Review of Clinical Trials." *Chin Med* doi: 10.1186/1749-8546-4-4 (2009)

68    Carr, D., and J. Lythgoe. "Use of Acupuncture during Labour." *Pract Midwife* 10th ser. 17.5 (2014): 12-15.

69  Manheimer, E., G. Zhang, L. Udoff, A. Haramati, et. al. "Effects of Acupuncture on Rates of Pregnancy and Live Birth among Women Undergoing in Vitro Fertilisation: Systematic Review and Meta-analysis." *BMJ* 336.7643 (2008): 545-49; Shuai, Z., F. Lian, P. Li, and W. Yang. "Effect of Transcutaneous Electrical Acupuncture Point Stimulation on Endometrial Receptivity in Women Undergoing Frozen-thawed Embryo Transfer: A Single-blind Prospective Randomised Controlled Trial." *Acupunct Med* 10 Oct 2014. Doi: 10.1136/acupubmed-2014-010572

70  Stener-Victorin, E., U. Waldenstrom, S. A. Andersson, and M. Wikland. "Reduction of Blood Flow Impedance in the Uterine Arteries of Infertile Women with Electro-acupuncture." *Hum Reprod* 11.6 (1996): 1314-317; Stener-Victorin, E., S. Fujisawa, and M. Kurosawa. "Ovarian Blood Flow Responses to Electroacupuncture Stimulation Depend on Estrous Cycle and on Site and Frequency of Stimulation in Anesthetized Rats." *J Appl Physiol* 101.1 (2006): 84-91.

71  Zhang, W.Y., G.Y. Huang, and J. Liu. "Influences of Acupuncture on Infertility of Rats with Polycystic Ovarian Syndrome." *Zhongguo Zhong Xi Yi Jie He Za Zhi* 29.11 (2009): 997-1000;
Shuai, Z., F. Lian, P. Li, and W. Yang. "Effect of Transcutaneous Electrical Acupuncture Point Stimulation on Endometrial Receptivity in Women Undergoing Frozen-thawed Embryo Transfer: A Single-blind Prospective Randomised Controlled Trial." *Acupunct Med* 10 Oct 2014. Doi: 10.1136/acupubmed-2014-010572.

72  Stener-Victorin, E., U. Waldenstrom, U. Tagnfors, T. Lundeberg, G. Lindstedt, and P. O. Janson. "Effects of Electro-acupuncture on Anovulation in Women with Polycystic Ovary Syndrome." *Acta Obstet Gynecol Scand* 79.3 (2000): 180-88.

73  Stener-Victorin, E., R. Kobayashi, O. Watanabe, T. Lundeberg, and M. Kurosawa. "Effect of Electro-acupuncture Stimulation of Different Frequencies and Intensities on Ovarian Blood Flow in Anaesthetized Rats with Steroid-induced Polycystic Ovaries." *Reprod Biol Endocrinol* 16th ser. 26.2 (2004).

74  Zhou, K., J. Jiang, J. Wu, and Z. Liu. "Electroacupuncture Modulates Reproductive Hormone Levels in Patients with Primary Ovarian Insufficiency: Results from a Prospective Observational Study." *Evid Based Complement Alternat Med* doi:10.1155.657234 (2013); Wang, F., Y. G. Fang, Y. R. Chen, and Et. Al. "Acupuncture for Premature Ovarian Failure: A Prospective Cohort Study." *Zhongguo Zhen Jiu* 34.7 (2014): 653-56.

75  Connor, B. "Compensatory Neurogenesis in the Injured Adult Brain." *Brain Injury: Pathogenesis, Monitoring, Recovery and Management*. Ed. A. Agrawal. Vol. doi: 10.5772/27004. InTech, 23 Mar. 2012; Leker, R.R., F. Soldner, I. Velasko, et. al. "Long-lasting Regeneration after Ischemia in the Cerebral Cortex."

*Stroke* 38.1 (2007): 153-61; Enciu, A.M., M.I. Nicolescu, C.G. Manole, et. al. "Neuroregeneration in Neurodegenerative Disorders." *BMC Neurology* 11.75 (2011); Jin, K., X. Wang, L. Xie, and Et. Al. "Evidence for Stroke-induced Neurogenesis in the Human Brain." *PNAS* 103.35 (2006): 13198-3202; Mu, Y., and F.H. Gage. "Adult Hippocampal Neurogenesis and Its Role in Alzheimer's Disease." *Molecular Neurodegeneration* 6.85 (2011).

[76] Doidge, Norman. *The Brain's Way of Healing: Remarkable Discoveries and Recoveries from the Frontiers of Neuroplasticity.* New York: Viking, 2015. Print.

[77] Nam, M.H., K.S. Ahn, and S.H. Choi. "Acupuncture Stimulation Induces Neurogenesis in Adult Brain." *Int Rev Neurobiol* 111 (2013): 67-90.

[78] Cho, S.Y., S.R. Shim, H.Y. Rhee, et. al. "Effectiveness of Acupuncture and Bee Venom Acupuncture in Idiopathic Parkinson's Disease." *Parkinsonism Relat Disord* 18.8 (2012): 948-52.; Shulman, L. M., X. Wen, W. J. Weiner, et. al. "Acupuncture Therapy for the Symptoms of Parkinson's Disease." *Mov Disord* 17.4 (2002): 799-802.

[79] Jeon, S., Y.J. Kim, S.T. Kim, et. al. "Proteomic Analysis of the Neuroprotective Mechanisms of Acupuncture Treatment in a Parkinson's Disease Mouse Model." *Proteonomics* 8.22 (2008): 4822-832.

[80] Kim, S.N., A.R. Doo, J.Y. Park, et. al. "Acupuncture Enhances the Synaptic Dopamine Availability to Improve Motor Function in a Mouse Model of Parkinson's Disease." *PLOS ONE*, 22 Nov. 2011.

[81] Xie, G., S. Yang, A. Chen, Z. Lin, et. al. "Electroacupuncture at Quchi and Zusanli Treats Cerebral Ischemia-reperfusion Injury through Activation of ERK Signaling." *Exp There Med* 5.6 (2013): 1593-597.

[82] Wang, Z., B. Nie, D. Li, Z. Zhao, and Et. Al. "Effect of Acupuncture in Mild Cognitive Impairment and Alzheimer Disease: A Functional MRI Study." Ed. XN Zuo. *PLOS ONE* 7.8 (2012): E42730.

[83] Zeng, Bai-Yun, Kaicun Zhao, and Fan-rong Liang. *Neurobiology of Acupuncture.* Vol. III. Oxford: Elsevier, 2013 p.129

[84] Cablioglu, M. T., and N. Ergene. "Changes in Levels of Serum Insulin, C-Peptide and Glucose after Electroacupuncture and Diet Therapy in Obese Women." *Am J Chin Med* 34.3 (2006): 367-76.

[85] Chang, S.L., J.G. Lin, T.C. Chi, I.M. Liu, and J.T. Cheng. "An Insulin-dependent Hypoglycaemia Induced by Electroacupuncture at the Zhongwan (CV12) Acupoint in Diabetic Rats." *Diabetologia* 42.2 (1999): 250-55.

[86] Ishizaki, N., N. Okushi, T. Yano, and Y. Yamamura. "Improvement in Glucose Tolerance as a Result of Enhanced Insulin Sensitivity during Electroacupuncture in Spontaneously Diabetic Goto-Kakizaki Rats." *Metabolism* 58.10 (2009): 1372-378.

[87] Fu, Shu-Ping, Su-Yun He, Bin Xu, Chen-Jun Hu, Sheng-Feng Lu, Wei-Xing Shen, Yan Huang, Hao Hong, Qian Li, Ning Wang, Xuan-Liang Liu,

Fanrong Liang, and Bing-Mei Zhu. "Acupuncture Promotes Angiogenesis after Myocardial Ischemia through H3K9 Acetylation Regulation at VEGF Gene." *PLOS ONE*. PLOS, 10 Apr. 2014.

## Chapter 6

[1] Langevin, H.M., and J.A. Yandow. "Relationship of Acupuncture Points and Meridians to Connective Tissue Planes." *The Anatomical Record* 269.6 (2002): 257-65.

[2] Manaka, Yoshio, Kazuko Itaya, and Stephen Birch. *Chasing the Dragon's Tail: The Theory and Practice of Acupuncture in the Work of Yoshio Manaka*. Brookline, MA: Paradigm Publications, 1995

[3] Chicurel, M.E., C.S. Chen, and D.E. Ingber. "Cellular Control Lies in the Balance of Forces." *Curr Opin Cell Biol* 10.2 (1998): 232-39; Chiquet, M. "Regulation of Extracellular Matrix Gene Expression by Mechanical Stress." *Matrix Biol* 18.5 (1999): 417-26.

[4] Bosman, F. T., and I. Stamenkovic. "Functional Structure and Composition of the Extracellular Matrix." *J Pathol* 200.4 (2003): 423-28.

[5] Findley, Thomas W. "Fascia Research from a Clinician/Scientist's Perspective." *Int J There Massage Bodywork* 4.4 (2011): 1-6.

[6] Langevin, H.M. "The Science of Stretch." *The Scientist*. LabX Media Group, 1 May 2013.

[7] Kwong, E.H., and T.W. Findley. "Journal of Rehabilitation Research & Development (JRRD)." *Journal of Rehabilitation Research* 51.6 (2014): 875-84. *Fascia-Current Knowledge and Future Directions in Physiatry: Narrative Review*. U.S. Department of Veterans Affairs.

[8] Ingber, D.E. "Cellular Mechanotransduction: Putting All the Pieces Together Again." *FASEB J* 20.7 (2006): 811-27.

[9] Langevin, H.M. "The Science of Stretch." *The Scientist*. LabX Media Group, 1 May 2013.

[10] Akst, Jef. "Full Speed Ahead." *The Scientist*. LabX Media Group, 1 Dec. 2009.

[11] Lipinski, B. "Biological Significance of Piezoelectricity in Relation to Acupuncture, Hatha Yoga, Osteopathic Medicine and Action of Air Ions." *Med Hypotheses* 3.1 (1977): 9-12; Oschman, James L. *Energy Medicine: The Scientific Basis*. Edinburgh: Churchill Livingstone, 2000.

[12] Becker, Robert O., and Gary Selden. *The Body Electric: Electromagnetism and the Foundation of Life*. New York: Morrow, 1985

[13] Maciocia, Giovanni. *The Channels of Acupuncture: Clinical Use of the Secondary Channels and Eight Extraordinary Vessels*. Edinburgh: Churchill Livingstone, 2006. P. 35

14    Maciocia, Giovanni. *The Channels of Acupuncture: Clinical Use of the Secondary Channels and Eight Extraordinary Vessels*. Edinburgh: Churchill Livingstone, 2006. pp. 46-50

15    Travell, Janet G., and David G. Simons. *Myofascial Pain and Dysfunction: The Trigger Point Manual*. Baltimore: Williams & Wilkins, 1983, ch. 49; Seem, Mark. *Acupuncture Physical Medicine: An Acupuncture Touchpoint Approach to the Treatment of Chronic Fatigue, Pain, and Stress Disorders*. Boulder, CO: Blue Poppy, 2000.

16    Langevin, H.M., and J.A. Yandow. "Relationship of Acupuncture Points and Meridians to Connective Tissue Planes." *The Anatomical Record* 269.6 (2002): 257-65.

17    Langevin, H.M. "The Science of Stretch." *The Scientist*. LabX Media Group, 1 May 2013

18    Langevin, H.M., D.L. Churchill, J. Wu, G.J. Badger, J.A. Yandow, J.R. Fox, and M.H. Krag. "Evidence of Connective Tissue Involvement in Acupuncture." *Faseb J.* 16 (2002): 872-74.

19    Langevin, H.M., and J.A. Yandow. "Relationship of Acupuncture Points and Meridians to Connective Tissue Planes." *The Anatomical Record* 269.6 (2002): 257-65.

20    Ahn, A. C., M. Park, J. R. Shaw, C. A. McManus, T. J. Kaptchuk, and H. M. Langevin. "Electrical Impedance of Acupuncture Meridians: The Relevance of Subcutaneous Collagenous Bands." *PLOS One* E11907 5.7 (2010)

21    Ingber, D.E. "The Architecture of Life." *Scientific American* 278.1 (1998): 48-57.

22    Guimberteau, Jean-Claude, M.D. "Endoscopy - Microvacuole - Surgeries Videos - Living Matter." DVD. *Surgery Videos - Living Matter, http://www. endovivo.com/en/dvds.php*

23    Moseley, J.B., et. al. "A Controlled Trial of Arthroscopic Surgery for Osteoarthritis of the Knee." *J Engl J Med* 347 (2002): 81-88.

## Chapter 7

1    Stuckey, H. L., and J. Nobel. "The Connection Between Art, Healing, and Public Health: A Review of Current Literature." *Am J Public Health* 100.2 (2010): 254-63.

2    NIH: National Center for Complementary and Alternative Medicine, http:// www.nlm.nih.gov/medlineplus/complementaryandalternativemedicine.html

3    Emanuel, Ezekiel J. "Why I Hope to Die at 75." *The Atlantic*. Atlantic Media Company, 17 Sept. 2014.

# INDEX

· · · · · · · · · · · · · · · · · · · · ·

Printed in the United States
By Bookmasters